PREFACE

An Alive Day within military references a day that is significant to the soldier as he/she should have been killed, but lived. An Alive Day is almost well known for Veterans as a national holiday. The idea is not to celebrate a severe injury or fellow military member deaths, but it is the individualistic celebration of life. The experience may range from an acute injury from a bomb blast to a bullet whipping past the head by inches. My Alive Day is September 8th, 2006. The machine gunner in a turret at the top of a gun truck is the most exposed person, and I was the gunner on September 8th, 2006, when a roadside bomb detonated immediately behind our truck. Black smoke and dust engulfed me. My immediate reaction was to duck, but since bending out of the way of an explosion is unlikely, I was more likely to be forced into the turret by the concussion blast. Please ring the chime as I suspected I was done.

The following thing I review is looking behind our truck, and seeing the dark tuft of smoke and my driver hollering at me on the headset on the off chance that I was alright. Inexplicably, I was not harmed. Past certain indications of a gentle blackout, I didn't have a scratch on me. The Afghan Army pickup truck that was closely following our firearm truck was not generally so fortunate as they got the immediate effect of the blast. The smell of the blast buildup was an appalling mix of cordite, consuming gas, and human tissue, and the equivocal smell of the Afghan residue. It was a smell that I can't satisfactorily portray and don't have any desire to smell again.

It is impossible to miss how a particular aroma can trigger recollections. The greater part of my recollections from my adolescence blurred throughout the long term. Notwithstanding, in the late spring, I could be driving past somebody trimming their grass, and the right blend of new cut grass and clover will in a flash put me at my grandma's home. I don't remember what year or how old I was or some other subtleties of the visit, however that unmistakable smell quickly ships me back on schedule. This blast smell is one that I never need openness to for the remainder of my life.

Upon reconnaissance of the scene, I saw a turned truck hood was lying on the contrary roadside where we had been. I was immersed in smoke and dust, and critical garbage things went right by me like shrapnel from a projectile. I can't clarify how I made due, not harmed, during this awful occasion past the Grace of God. Consistently, on September eighth, I

email the driver of our weapon truck to wish him, "Cheerful Alive Day!" I had a few other near calamities and horrible mishaps, yet this day stands apart from the rest.

PART ONE

UNIQUE COMBAT DEPLOYMENT AS A COMBAT ADVISOR

INTRODUCTION

"Give a man a fish and feed him for a day. Encourage a man to fish and take care of him for a lifetime" – Chinese Proverb

The Islamic Republic of Afghanistan is a landlocked country in South-Central Asia. Pakistan borders it in the south and east, Iran in the west, and Turkmenistan, Uzbekistan, Tajikistan, and China in the north. Nicknamed the "Cemetery of Empires," Afghanistan has an extremely long history of military missions by Alexander the Great, Mongols, British, Soviets, and the US. Afghanistan's capital, Kabul, has an expected populace of 3,000,000 individuals, and practically 80% of the Afghan populace lives in country regions with no other city in excess of 500,000 individuals. Afghanistan is around the size of the State of Texas and is generally a similar scope. Afghanistan contains deserts in the south (800 feet above ocean level) to the beginning of the Hindu Kush Mountains in the upper east (24,000 feet above ocean level) and is by and large a parched climate. The temperatures can go from under zero degrees Fahrenheit in the colder time of year to in excess of 120 degrees Fahrenheit in the summer.

Operation Enduring Freedom was the authority name of the US military mission against the Global War on Terrorism. Because of the assaults on September eleventh, 2001, the US started airstrikes in Afghanistan against Al Qaeda and the Taliban on October seventh, 2001. By the start of November, the US Special Forces and the Northern Alliance, well disposed Afghan local army, battled against the Taliban and dealt with the majority of the country. Osama Bin Laden and his Al Qaeda association utilized Afghanistan for preparing bases; notwithstanding, the gossip is that Osama Bin Laden pulled out to Pakistan during the Battle of Tora Bora in December 2001. Numerous other commanders

and sub-authorities remained, and alongside huge number of unfamiliar contenders and Taliban.

In December 2004, Hamid Karzai was chosen as the primary president, and the Afghanistan National Army was quickly standing up. The US powers, for the most part in the east, centered around battling psychological militants or preparing the Afghan Army and helped with the Afghan Army development. Indeed, even with 23,000 US fighters in Afghanistan in 2006, numerous units and troops were under-resourced. The Afghanistan war was alluded to as "the other conflict" as the military and principle political exertion zeroed in on Operation Iraqi Freedom. In 2006, the US had 88 setbacks with a sharp expansion in side of the road bombs. Notwithstanding the fights and adversary dangers, there were great many extra mines from the Soviet intrusion undermining troops and civilians.

In 2003, Combined Joint Task Force Phoenix shaped Embedded Training Teams, or battle counsels, utilizing tenth Mountain Division warriors and thoughtfully utilizes regular powers to prepare and coach Afghan soldiers. The wide battle guide's main goal is to exhort the Afghan Army in initiative, staff support capacities, arranging, evaluating, supporting, and executing activities and preparing. Battle consultants additionally give the Afghan Army admittance to close air support, field big guns backing, and clinical clearing as battle empowering influences. The roughly 6,000 individuals from Task Force Phoenix end objective was to have the Afghan Army and Afghan police to be independent to work without alliance assistance.

From 2003 through 2006, the preparation for battle guides was not normalized, and preparing was at various establishments around the US. In October 2006, all the groundwork for battle guides was united at Fort Riley, Kansas, with a standard preparing program. The battle counselor is definitely not a doctrinal unit or mission and is a greater amount of the mission subset of the Special Forces to prepare an unfamiliar inner guard. Be that as it may, Special Forces get long periods of preparing to be completely qualified while the preparation for battle guides was under a month and a half. The battle counselor didn't have committed assets like Special Forces and needed to depend on presents from customary powers. Team Phoenix in the long run disbanded in 2010 with the foundation of NATO Training Mission-Afghanistan. Several exceptionally perceived battle counsels are Captain William Swenson and Corporal Dakota Meyer. They got the Medal of Honor for their activities during the Battle of Ganjgal in 2009.

Being a battle consultant was far beyond being a tutor or being

in a homeroom, and the obligations frequently differed between organization levels and corps levels. With my sending cycle and various tasks, I encountered the full range of activities, from the overall security in Gardez to living in a weapon truck for north of seven days. My arrangement was not with a natural or customary unit, as I filled an opportunity inside a set up team. I had four tasks on three distinct bases, moving practical regions from signal, to infantry, to handle big guns. Overall, just 0.4% of the American populace is in the military, and an expected 7.3% of all living Americans have served in the military eventually in their lives. Not all tactical faculty convey or have sent into an antagonistic nation, and one more little rate were engaged with battle activities. Roughly 28% of the sent powers were battle centered, while the leftover 72% zeroed in on coordinations, life backing, organization, and base camp. Accordingly, being a field cannons official conveyed to Afghanistan as a battle guide in 2006 was truly unique.

Combat Advisor Staffing

HQ/ 2nd IN Bde/ 203 IN Corps			
	01	LTC	BDE TEAM CHIEF
	02	SGM	CSM MENTOR / NCOIC
	03	MAJ	BDE XO / ORD OFF
	04	MAJ	OPS / INTEL OFF
	05	SFC	OPS NCO
	06	MAJ	PERS / LOG OFF
	07	SFC	ADMIN / LOG NCO
	08	CPT	OPS / INTEL OFF
	09	CPT	FIELD ARTY OFF
	10	CPT	SIGNAL OFF
	11	SFC	COMMO NCO
	12	CPT	MED OFF
	13	SFC	MED NCO
	14	CPT	MOTOR OFF
	15	SPC	SUPPLY / DRIVER
	16	SPC	CLERK / DRIVER

Battalion

HQ/ 4th CS Bn/ 2nd IN Bde / 203 IN Corps			
	01	MAJ	BN TEAM CHIEF
	02	CPT	OPS / INTEL OFF
	03	CPT	PERS / LOG OFF
	04	CPT	MOTOR OFF
	05	MSG	OPS NCO / CSM MENTOR
	06	SFC	NCO MENTOR
Co A/ 4th CS Bn/ 2nd IN Bde / 203 IN Corps			
	07	CPT	CO TEAM CHIEF
	08	SFC	CO NCO MENTOR
Co B/ 4th CS Bn/ 2nd IN Bde / 203 IN Corps			
	09	CPT	CO TEAM CHIEF
	10	SFC	CO NCO MENTOR
Co C/ 4th CS Bn/ 2nd IN Bde / 203 IN Corps			
	11	CPT	CO TEAM CHIEF
	12	SFC	CO NCO MENTOR
Co D/ 4th CS Bn/ 2nd IN Bde / 203 IN Corps			
	13	CPT	CO TEAM CHIEF
	14	SFC	CO NCO MENTOR
HHC/ 4th CS Bn/ 2nd IN Bde / 203 IN Corps			
	15	CPT	CO TEAM CHIEF
	16	SFC	CO NCO MENTOR

Brigade

★★★★ US Central Command

★★★ Combined Forces Command – Afghanistan

★★ Combined Security Transition Command – Afghanistan

★ Combined Joint Task Force Phoenix

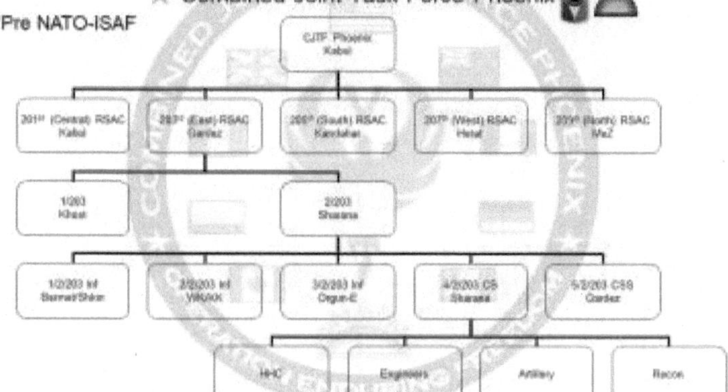

203rd Corps Spring Stationing

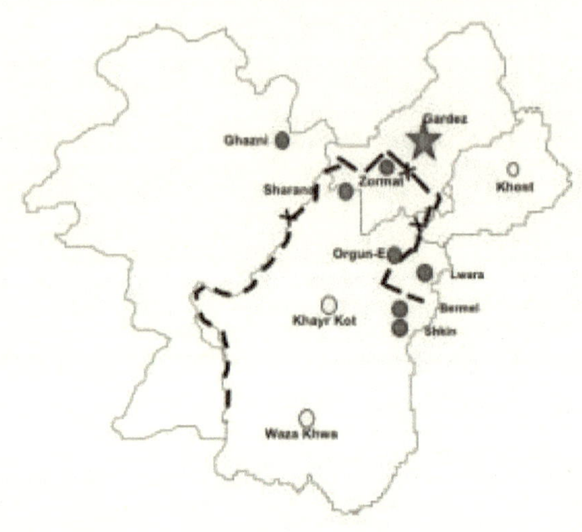

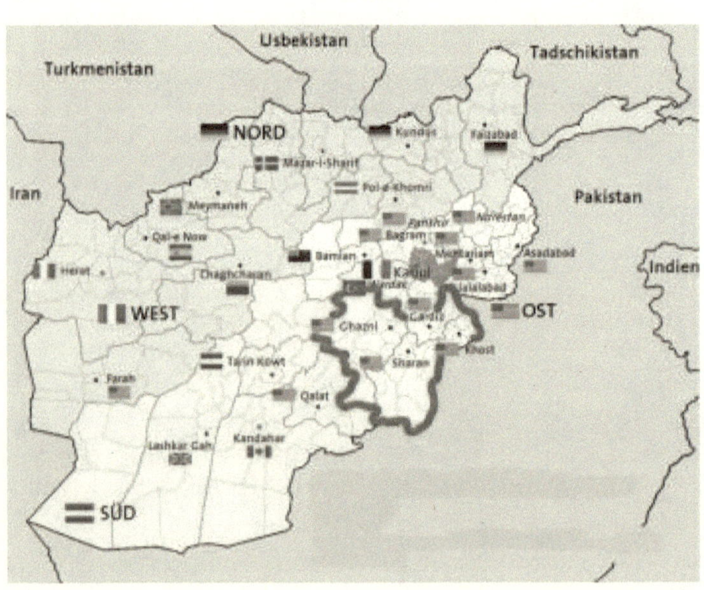

WHERE ARE WE GOING?

"Where'd who go?" – Top Gun

In the fall of 2005, I was an active status as a Captain assigned as the brigade fire control officer in the Wisconsin National Guard. The week before Thanksgiving in 2005, I received a phone call from the brigade leader asking on the off chance that I was keen on sending with him for an implanted preparing group mission to Afghanistan. I would come to discover that an implanted preparing group was usually truncated to ETT. Toward the start of Operation Enduring Freedom, the military was entrusted to build up and train the military in Afghanistan, and the installed preparing group idea created. The implanted preparing group name was explicit to Afghanistan tasks, and Iraq activities had comparative groups with the name of Military Transition Teams, or MiTTs. The conventional name of the battle counsel would be more fitting, like the battle guides during the Vietnam War.

I knew very little with regards to Afghanistan for sure the mission would involve. To me, I thought I was venturing out from home for a year to a weird spot to be some sort of teacher. Around then, my significant other and I encountered hardships beginning a family, and we were presently fruitfulness specialist visits. I let the unit authority in on that it was not the best planning in view of this issue. On that Monday morning, the second-in-order informed me that both he and I would prepare toward the start of January 2006. I would have a little more than a month, which included two significant occasions to get ready. Basically with Thanksgiving and Christmas, I would have the chance to see all my relatives. I discovered that my task was a transmission official since I had an essential information on radios, signal working instructions,

PCs, and networking.

Almost four years earlier, I was the preparation official in a field ordnance contingent. On September eleventh, 2001, I headed to work and heard on the radio with regards to a plane colliding with the World Trade Center in New York City. I felt that it more likely than not been an awful pilot to hit such a huge structure. Soon after I showed up, I was called to the field big guns unit base camp as they had a TV and was showing the subsequent accident. We were coordinated into a lock-down and kept up with responsibility. The brigade official in-control was on leave visiting his family in the State of Washington, and he discovered that he was stuck there as every one of the trips the nation over were grounded. I needed to accept control of the staff and our far off units. I spent the remainder of that day in our work force office as they had a TV. We watched the pinnacles fall, and the plane accidents at the Pentagon and Pennsylvania and the persistent media inclusion attempting to sort out what was happening.

I have been keen on serving in the military since the time joining the Tiger Cubs and Boy Scouts and playing G.I. Joe toys. At my Eagle Scout grant function in Boy Scouts, I had a ceremonial group from a nearby Reserve Officer Training Corps (ROTC) present the National Colors. During the initial not many long stretches of secondary school, my fantasy was to turn into an Army helicopter pilot, and I read Robert Mason's Chickenhawk (1983), a few times. At the point when I was 16 years of age, I discovered that my vision precluded me for flight, and my decision of life moved into the US Marine Corps. I was genuinely considering the postponed passage program.

When I was 17 years of age and working in the café in my little old neighborhood in focal Wisconsin, I wound up talking with a benefactor enrollment specialist for the Army National Guard. He persuaded me to join, and I enrolled under the split-choice program, which empowered me to finish fundamental preparing the late spring after my lesser year of secondary school and my high level cannons preparing the late spring after graduation. I was guileless to the tactical way of life, so the low maintenance viewpoint was engaging as I could go to school and have a vocation while serving my country. In 1993, I had no clue about where my tactical profession would go and how world occasions would wind up sending me most of the way all over the planet into fight. At that point, I had no clue about what the field cannons did or how it was organized. My spotter said this was a cool occupation since it included lasers and computers.

I went to my fundamental preparing in 1993 at Fort Leonardwood,
Missouri, and

was with Sergeant First Class Crider and Sergeant First Class Lyons as my drill educators. The gossip is valid that you always remember your drill teachers. The accompanying summer, I finished my high level mounted guns preparing as the honor graduate in Fort Sill. I partook in my high level preparing, not just in light of the fact that I did well with the topic, yet additionally with the expectation of complimentary time on the ends of the week. Frequently a gathering of us would bring a taxi into Lawton simply past the fundamental door to the clubs. There were around four or five clubs in succession, and the talk was that our First Sergeant was part proprietor of one of the clubs. These clubs were notable for not actually looking at ID, and our gathering of 18-year-olds wound up spending a lot of cash on refreshments and diversion, all under the lawful drinking age.

I got the epithet "Chickenhawk" rapidly as a size reference with the chickenhawk in the Looney Tunes animation, Foghorn Leghorn. The epithet stuck for a long time, and I preferred the linkage with one of my beloved books. I was exceptionally anxious to take on different obligations and did well progress of time party tasks, getting ready for the fundamental unit to show up. I turned into the essential vehicle driver of an enormous followed garrison and the auxiliary PC operator.

I met my future spouse first year of school, and we began dating on and off. Proposing to turn into an Army official, I started to investigate the ROTC program at Marquette University. I pursued military science second semester and applied for a three-year grant. Toward the finish of my first year, ROTC granted me a grant. Nonetheless, I had not involved myself in scholastics, and ROTC promptly pulled out the grant offer. I proceeded with ROTC in an exceptional program, which would keep me in the official preparing pipeline and keep on boring with my National Guard unit. After my sophomore year, I moved to the University of Wisconsin – Milwaukee because of monetary reasons and still lived at Marquette University to proceed with Marquette University ROTC. Throughout the spring field preparing exercise in April 1997 at Fort McCoy, Wisconsin, I separated my kneecap while getting around a log during an attack on a fortification. My treatment incorporated a support and non-weight holding on for bolsters for half a month, so participation at ROTC progressed camp in Fort Lewis, Washington, was sketchy. Luckily, I had the option to recuperate enough before I left in August. This injury would cause issues down the road for me later in my profession as there was huge ligament damage.

moved on from the University of Wisconsin - Milwaukee and received

my bonus as a subsequent lieutenant in May 1998. I had a serene summer functioning as a safety officer in the Grand Avenue Mall in Milwaukee and went to my Field Artillery Officer Basic Course in Fort Sill in August 1998. With my field gunnery preparing and encounters from the past five years, this five-drawn out course was a breeze, and I graduated with distinction on the Commandant's List. There was a gathering of around six of us that were in every case together. Regularly, the others would carry brew to my quarters as a motivator to assist them with their schoolwork. Perhaps the best part of this course was that most understudies dwelled in a tall structure in rooms like a little lodging. Interestingly, few us lived in two-story structures like lofts with a different room, lounge, washroom, and a common kitchen with every day house cleaner administration. Our gathering would invest free energy on the official's green, for the most part hitting the balls for fun.

My significant other and I wedded in 2001 and claimed a house in south-focal Wisconsin, and she worked for the region in adolescent social work. I feared informing my better half regarding my organization. I generally understood that a sending may be conceivable, particularly after the 9/11 assaults, however never figured it would happen to me. My significant other and I were agreeable without anyone else, and we're attempting to begin a family. We didn't have a broad social encouraging group of people as both our folks lived just about two hours away, and we were not near any of our neighbors. I struggled attempting to envision what I would be going through over the course of the following year, and I had a much harder time attempting to envision what my better half or family would be going through.

The main day of assembly was on January fifth, 2006, and was my 30th birthday celebration. We had a short gathering to get to know one another. Our Wisconsin guide bunch comprised of 16 work force, half officials, and half sergeants, with an underlying task to an Afghanistan National Army unit base camp. I chipped away at event with a couple of the officials, yet I didn't know the greater part of them. The officers in our gathering came from all over the state and diverse units.

The following several days were family briefings and individual hardware confrontations, and ensuring we each had the right number of bottles, hiking beds, and other gear. The third day was an enthusiastic farewell function and bidding farewell to my relatives and spouse. I had the option to get my five seconds of distinction during a meeting with the neighborhood news after the service. We changed into regular citizen garments and loaded up the transport to go to the air terminal for a business trip to Mississippi.

There were four detachment level and five brigade level consultant groups from different states going through this emphasis of preparation preparing. We lived in lofts in a substantial square sleeping quarters working with another state's counsel group on the opposite side. The bathrooms were a few structures away, and the encompassing region had an eating office, clothing trailers, and a little shoppette around a five-minute leave. We actually utilized individual mobile phones, and I had the option to call home pretty much consistently as there was negligible internet.

he climate at Camp Shelby was significantly hotter contrasted with Wisconsin in January and February. It was adequately cold to wear whimper gear, similar to polypropylene and long clothing, to keep warm, and we needed to wear our downy coats incidentally. The majority of the preparation was nonexclusive by going to classes, going to rifle ranges, becoming battle lifeline qualified, and finishing land route courses. We had some Afghanistan and battle counsel explicit preparing, which was for the most part defective. We had a class on the strategic satellite radio however didn't have any satellite time portion to utilize the radios. We had Dari language classes on a few nights yet wound up in the Pashto talking region. The greater part of the educators continued to allude to Iraq, which was an alternate battle climate than Afghanistan. I liked the preparation on unfamiliar weapons, for example, the AK-47 attack rifle, PKM automatic weapon, and Dragunov marksman rifle.

We went through uniform fittings for the new designed regalia and tan softened cowhide boots, and I was happy that I held off buying the new garbs ahead of time. We went through the quick handling drive that gave the most recent stuff, like the protective cap, new designed pockets, shades, and goggles. The body protection that was given was the tan desert design, and with estimating issues and rainchecks, the whole gathering of counsels had portions of each of the three uniform examples. Towards the finish of the preparation time frame, practically the entirety of our stuff was in the new example; nonetheless, our body covering was as yet a desert design. One person in our gathering was worried about being an objective with various examples. He bought extra new example coats and had a nearby designer utilize the material to make another cover for his body protective layer. It was only two or three days after he got his cover when we were completely given new designed covers for our body shield. We regularly reprimanded him in light of his additional buys, like two or three hundred-dollar electric lamp, an exorbitant blade to just be utilized close by to-hand battle, custom options to his rifle, and his humongous lawn seat. Normal military vernacular would allude to him as

a geardo.

verall, I felt that we were preparing to prepare and actually take a look at the cases as opposed to planning for war. During this time span in the conflict, customary Army organizations were for a considerable length of time. The 365-day organization time would not begin until appearance in the theater, so the time at Camp Shelby would be extra preparing time away from home. Different administrations and associations had their arrangement cycles, for example, the ordinary three-month revolution for Air Force staff. Ultimately, most regular Army arrangements were for quite some time with two or three months for training.

ENEMY FORCES

"The foe of my adversary is my companion" – Arabic Proverb

The most significant difference between modern warfare and world wars is that the enemy does not wear a uniform. The simple act of putting a uniform on makes it so much easier to define the enemy. The soldiers in World War Two may have unexpectedly walked into an ambush along a dirt road, but they had the opportunity to fight back. Our military has a significant disadvantage as we bring the fight in our uniforms to a faraway land to fight the unknown, strictly following the laws of war.

We received the laws of war briefing from the Army lawyers, which outlines when you may fire your weapon. If an enemy fired at us, we could shoot back for self-defense. There may be situations where you may initiate fire upon someone if there was a specific threat and had hostile actions. An example is a military-age male picking up a rocket-propelled grenade and getting ready to fire at your approaching convoy. Unfortunately, there are too many different situations to cover what may be allowed or considered a war crime. This vagueness created uncertainty as you wanted to protect yourself and others; however, no one wanted to end up in prison for committing a war crime by breaking the rules.

he AK-47 Kalashnikov is a 7.62mm assault rifle. It is the most popular and widely used assault rifle in the world, used by the Afghan Army, Afghan Police, Romanian advisors, and the enemy. An AK-47 assault rifle wouldn't automatically identify a person as an enemy. The Afghan Police didn't always have a uniform, so it would be common to see a male with an AK-47 standing at an intersection in a town.

Afghanistan is an asymmetric battlespace, and the enemy doesn't wear a uniform or follow the Geneva Convention rules. The enemy consisted of the Haqqani network, Taliban, Al Qaida, foreign fighters, local warlords, and others from more than 20 various enemy organizations. We generally grouped the enemy and referred to them as anti-coalition forces. It is common to see a military-age male appearing to be working in the farm field to support his family one minute, and then triggering a roadside bomb the next moment, and pick up his shovel again. Our military could not engage the male unless we saw a hostile act. Most of the enemy knows our rules and that we follow the rules, and they use this to their advantage. Most combat environments have an offense and defense, and asymmetrical warfare always put us on the defense.

The general enemy pattern was to move into Pakistan over the winter months because the snow in the mountains prohibited practical travel. The enemy used the winter months to recover and to train. Once enough snow melted in the spring, the enemy began the spring offensive and fighting season by moving into Afghanistan. The enemy conducted their attacks against Afghan and coalition forces through the summer and then traveled back to Pakistan in the late fall. We could expect a few attacks during the winter from left behind forces or local forces, but the attacks were significantly less than the summertime.

As a combat advisor, especially at the company level, I was not included in enemy threat briefings, targeting meetings, or decision on combat operations. I was at the tactical level, executing our specific missions and wouldn't understand who the enemy was until we were engaged. Our advisor teams did not have any intelligence capabilities, nor did we receive any intelligence reports from nearby friendly forces. Almost all of the intelligence that I heard about came from word of mouth by the Afghan Army and local government elders.

One of the most substantial obstacles from obtaining intelligence from local Afghans is that no one could be trusted. With blatant corruption and tribal feuds, there was no way to determine the truth. There are numerous attempts of an Afghan reporting that another Afghan planted a roadside bomb, but the first Afghan is seeking revenge for a long-time tribal fight.

n 2006, the enemy used roadside bomb attacks very commonly in Iraq, and this method of attack increased dramatically in Afghanistan. A roadside bomb is an explosive, from a hand-made pipe bomb to a large artillery round. Roadside bombs can be detonated by different means, ranging from pressure plates to wired to cell phones. We received training on identifying roadside bombs, but this was very difficult in Afghanistan as almost all the roads were dirt, and there was garbage all over the place. Most of the gun trucks had electronic counter-measures installed, which would interfere with radio and some cell phone signals. However, this interference was limited in space around the gun truck and wouldn't affect roadside bombs with pressure plates or wires.

or the three weeks that I was at Bermel, we experienced 11 rocket attacks. I only kept track of the rocket attacks with impacts inside of the outer perimeter, and there wasn't an attack with less than six rockets. One of the rocket attacks had 21 rockets. The rocket attacks started as a nuisance but quickly changed into real danger with injuries, and an Afghan Army soldier killed in his bunk when a rocket impacted his quarters. You feel helpless during a rocket attack because you don't know where they will land or how many there will be, and you can't do anything but seek cover and hope that a rocket doesn't impact next to you. The first couple of attacks, my sergeant advisor, Ressler, and I ran to the Marine combat advisor building for cover, but since it wasn't our building, we were in the way by standing around in the hallway. We decided that it would be safe to use our gun truck for cover as it should stop any shrapnel.

Additionally, we could turn the radio onto the Task Force Catamount net to listen to the updates from the operations center and the artillery sections to give us better situational awareness. Our gun truck stopped some shrapnel as a rocket impacted within yards of us. A piece of shrapnel put a hole in our gun truck hood about the size of a half pencil but didn't appear to damage anything in the engine compartment. Another piece of shrapnel put a small crack and chip in the passenger side windshield, right where I was sitting. The bulletproof windshield stopped the shrapnel and looked similar to medium-sized stone damage from highway driving in a standard car. The damage wasn't significant, but the windshield would have to be replaced to maintain the protection's integrity. One Task Force Wolfpack soldier was wounded on his hand from shrapnel during one rocket attack, and an Afghan Army artillery soldier incurred a small head wound from shrapnel in another rocket attack. One rocket landed in the construction yard and started a small fire.

Being on the receiving end of incoming rocket fires creates a huge psychosis effect that instills a tremendous, helpless fear. In the first half of my deployment, I learned and responded that the enemy has limited quantities of rockets, and they were notorious for being inaccurate. I was in two separate rocket attacks when I was in Gardez, each with only one rocket. When I was in Bermel, things were drastically different. During the first couple of attacks, I still had the mindset of inaccuracy and a nuisance. The general attitude was that the enemy would have to be very lucky, and it was just your time as the chance of being struck by lightning was greater. As soon as we started receiving at least six rockets in our perimeter almost every other day, there was nothing more than I wanted to hide or go away.

Bermel had a radar system that could detect incoming rockets and provide the fire direction center the grid coordinates to shoot back; however, the radar could only detect 107mm rockets as the 122mm rockets had a lower flight path. There wasn't a prominent voice in the sky or an alarm for incoming rockets like some of the more massive bases. Messages went across the radio nets, and everybody started yelling and running for cover. If the rocket impacted nearby, you could hear the short whistle sound. If the rocket impacted close, it was just an explosion sound without the whistle. Task Force Wolfpack almost always fired rounds at the launch points for counter-fire. Still, the enemy usually had the rockets set on timers, so there was no enemy personnel in the area. There was a time or two with a subsequent explosion report, which indicated that the counter-fire likely destroyed new rockets waiting to fire. Occasionally, air support was available, and Air Force B-1 Lancer or F-16 Fighting Falcon dropped smart bombs onto the rocket launch sites. Even from several miles away at the base, you could hear the impact and see the smoke clouds from these massive explosions.

Bermel also had a Joint Land Elevated Netted Sensor System (JLENS) for additional observation beyond the machine gun towers. The JLENS was a high-tech camera on a tall tower with day and infrared full-motion video cameras with impressive zooming capabilities. From the computer system in the operations center, you could operate the camera's direction and zoom and obtain grid coordinates. Depending on the rocket attack's launch spot, the JLENS could be used to see the counter-fire effects. I would use the JLENS to observe our Afghan Army artillery fires because the Afghan Army didn't have trained observers.

EVERYDAY LIFE

"If you have more than what you need, build a longer table, not a higher fence." - Unknown

BASES

Generally, there are two types of bases: the US and the Afghan Army. Task Force Catamount operated most of the US bases in our area with their infantry units and their provincial reconstruction teams. Combat advisors resided in a separate section on Afghan Army bases. Gardez and Sharana were Afghan Army bases, and Bermel was a US base on one half and Afghan Army on the other, and Task Force Catamount controlled the whole base.

Most of the bases I resided where located on the outskirts of the town, with an outer wire perimeter and a HESCO barrier wall inner perimeter with one main entry point for vehicles. The unit controlling the base would provide security at the entry gate, and the machine guns in the watchtowers around the inner perimeter. HESCO barriers are mainly large sandbags used to construct perimeter walls to protect from projectiles and explosions. A HESCO barrier is made from fabric lined, wire woven cubes that engineering equipment fills with sand and dirt. Two soldiers and a front loader can construct ten yards of a HESCO barrier wall in 20 minutes; the same size wall built with sandbags would take eight soldiers eight hours. HESCO barriers are available in various heights, widths, and lengths, and they can be stacked to additional heights. The HESCO perimeter walls would completely obstruct the surrounding view from inside the walls; therefore, there is an essential requirement to establish armed watchtowers.

All the bases had a variety of living, bathrooms, and dining buildings. The majority of the buildings on the bases were B-Huts. Local construction workers made the B-Huts of cheap 2x4s and plywood with a metal roof. The approximate 150 square foot structure had a plywood floor and plexiglass windows that were boarded up to restrict light from escaping. There was a smattering of concrete buildings on the bases that generally housed soldiers and the operations center. However, the concrete did not meet the US standards for concrete and would likely not survive a direct hit from enemy weapons or rockets. The concrete would resist shrapnel much better than plywood. Shipping containers are a common sight around the base. Shipping containers are mostly used for storage of cases of water, spare parts, and extra equipment. A variety of shipping containers are retrofitted to be a bathroom or a small living area for several soldiers.

Large generators created electrical power for the bases and continuously ran at a high decibel level. Generators produce unreliable 220-volt power, and you needed to acquire a power converter to downgrade to the American standard 110 volts for our computers, printers, and other usual devices. These large generators needed to be shut down for routine maintenance and would occasionally break down completely, resulting in no electrical power.

Males dominated the large bases and were the sole gender at small bases. 2006 was before the integration of females in a combat unit and combat jobs; however, females indeed deployed to Iraq and Afghanistan in support. Rocket attacks or roadside bombs do not discriminate based on gender or any other protected classes, and females were in convoys and resided on some bases. There were no females in Sharana or Bermel as these were small bases with only combat soldiers. Gardez has about a half dozen females, and Camp Phoenix had a much more significant percentage. The smaller bases also did not have the structures or capabilities to support separated living areas and bathrooms. In contrast, Camp Phoenix had several designated B-huts for living areas and trailers for bathrooms.

AGRAM

Bagram is a super base, with the coalition headquarters elements, contractors, cargo aircraft, fighter aircraft, helicopters, and the primary logistics center. The main road at Bagram, Disney Drive, divides the base, with the Air Force and Army aviation, medical and operations center on one side and the other side with the dining facility, shoppette, barracks, and other

amenities. The gym facility is in a colossal clamshell tent near the center of the base. The shoppette is relatively large, and there are several other eating options outside, such as Burger King and a pizza place. The additional great comfort at Bagram is the USO building, where popcorn is always available and shows movies. Transit soldiers, like myself, slept on a metal bunk bed in a darkened tent. Personnel assigned to Bagram would be very similar to a US installation in the states. The Military Police conducted law enforcement operations for speeding, and contractors provided laundry service. The size and assets available drastically reduced the number of attacks on the base, so it was considered a safe zone.

CAMP PHOENIX

Camp Phoenix would be considered a large base and was on the eastern side of Kabul, surrounded in a semi-urban environment. Camp Phoenix is a US base with several hundred occupants with Task Force Phoenix's headquarters and elements of the foreign advisor teams. Near the front of the camp was a small two-story shoppette building with a small barbershop, a famous Green Bean coffee shop, a Dairy Queen ice cream shop, a pizza shop, and a small shoppette. Subway restaurant had a van parked outside the shoppette doors; however, the sandwiches didn't look quite right. Near the shoppette was the library and the gym, and the best part of the gym was that they kept the popcorn machine full. I never made it past the popcorn machine. A large contracting company operated a large dining facility, and the food was all right.

The finance office was located by the dining facility and was the only place to cash a check or exchange dollars for Afghani currency. Camp Phoenix had its fire department with a military fire truck and a chapel that provided services for several dominations and languages. On the south side of the base was a large, oval running track, and the inside of the running track was a helicopter landing zone.

GARDEZ

The medium-size Gardez base is situated on the southeast side of Gardez, and there are two small hills to the east, and there is a small mountain on the north side of the base. The Afghan base size is roughly three city blocks by three city blocks, with the US advisor portion occupying one block. The rest of the area contained barracks, officer quarters, dining facility, medical, headquarters buildings, maintenance buildings, and parking areas for about 1,000 Afghan Army soldiers.

The advisor portion had its perimeter and entry gate, corps headquarters building, a dining facility operated by contractors, a fitness room, a small medical clinic, a maintenance area, and a large parking area. The entire advisor compound was covered in gravel to reduce the moon dust and had sidewalks installed along the row of B-Huts. Walking across the gravel became very annoying very quickly.

SHARANA

Sharana was approximately 7,000 ft. in elevation, and the surrounding area was arid with very little vegetation, dry river beds, some farm fields, and mud-walled Afghan homes. About the size of a city block, the Afghan base supported about 250 combat support Afghan Army soldiers and was in the stages of bringing in the Afghan Army brigade headquarters. The US personnel had an inner compound surrounded by HESCOs that was roughly the size of a football field.

The sleeping quarters were made of bricks with a slightly reinforced plywood roof and had two or three rooms per building and three or four persons per room. The room closest to the restroom was designed as the operations center and contained a couple of computers, standard team equipment, and an extensive planning table. Around the corner of our operations center was a small HESCO bunker. The general layout of the advisor base was a horizontal "T," with the top of thr "T" being the restroom and the sleeping quarters along the base of the "T" across from each other, creating a mini alleyway.

Two gates separated the US compound from the Afghan Army compound. We kept the smaller gate unlocked to allow access to the interpreters. The more massive metal gate was kept closed and locked with a combination padlock, which we would have to open up every time we took the gun trucks. The Afghan Army soldiers operated the main entry gate to the base and manned watchtowers around the perimeter. Electric power came from the generator located immediately behind the row of sleeping quarters. The combat support advisors were the primary US personnel, and there were a Task Force Catamount representative and a few contractors for the district governor. There were approximately two to three dozen US personnel total.

BERMEL

Bermel was a small Task Force Catamount base with a US infantry company and an Afghan Army battalion. Bermel is situated in a flat valley and is roughly the size of a skinny city block. The mountains and surrounding areas had trees and greens among the rough rocks. The base was divided roughly in half, one side for the US and one side for the Afghan Army. Task Force Catamount occupied the US side with the Marine combat advisors. The buildings were mostly concrete and had a few B-Huts for contractors and transients. The US side had concrete watchtowers, operations center, barracks, dining facility, gym, medics, maintenance bays, fuel bladders, two 105mm howitzers, and a radar. The Afghan Army side consisted of mostly brick buildings for barracks, a dining facility, and a small parking area. The main gate for the base was on the Afghan Army side with a small medical clinic and the local Afghan district center. Staying in Bermel is like living in the Wild West.

COMMUNICATIONS

When I reference the radio, I am referring to encrypted tactical radios with call signs. No radio station played top 40 music hits or a Paul Harvey story.

There was spotty coverage of local Afghan radio stations that the Afghan soldiers listened to, but if I wanted to listen to music, I would need my Palm Pilot or an iPod. The tactical radios had a range of a few miles but often was limited due to terrain. Some of the tactical radios could connect via satellite, which was needed for convoys as the bases were too spread out for tactical radios. If the combat advisors required to talk to each other in a convoy or back to the base, we needed to use the tactical radios.

Every one of the guide groups was likewise alluded to by their call signs. A detachment or corps staff officials had call signs assigned, however they normally don't utilize the radios. The names and call signs are significantly more common at the legion and friends levels. The unit consultant group's call sign was "Seminole," the call sign for the Romanian force guide group was "Vampire," and the battle support legion counsel's call sign was "Blackfoot." Traditionally, number six of a consider sign recognizes the administrator, and numeral seven of a call sign assigns the sergeant-in-control. My call sign in the Afghan Army first Infantry Battalion was "Vampire 1" as I was the work force official. My call sign in the battle support regiment was "Blackfoot 36," showing that I was responsible for the third organization. Call finishes paperwork for all units and associations in Afghanistan are overseen at the Combined Forces Command – Afghanistan level to quickly

distinguish whom you are conversing with on the radio.

Internet and phone associations shift on the spot, with most huge bases having wired associations and more modest bases utilizing little satellite associations. A portion of the enormous bases depended on the tactical phone framework and could call military telephones in the US. To settle on a decision home, we would have to utilize the telephone place or a tactical phone to dial an administrator at the nearest army base in the US. Then, at that point, you needed to request to be moved to a 800 distinguishing mark number, and afterward have the option to dial home and be charged on the calling card from the establishment to the house. There were 15 minutes time limits on the telephones, which you could scarcely see one another or would cut off totally, subsequent to sitting tight in line for 30-45 minutes. It was extremely disappointing to dial the long numbers to arrive at the US establishment, the calling card 800 number, and the full home number to be cut off. Obviously, there is no security as you are sitting right close to another person, and individuals in line are in a rush to get their turn.

I at last purchased an Afghan wireless for about $100 and afterward purchased telephone cards to stack minutes into my record, which worked out to be around $0.45/min to call home. The PDA functioned admirably around Gardez for periodic, short calls. The phone inclusion outside Gardez and Kabul diminished significantly with the absence of pinnacles and the always present mountains.

The little puts together depended with respect to a little satellite for telephone and web associations. These satellites were little and just upheld two telephone lines and four web lines. The telephones were not on the tactical organization, so we were unable to utilize them to call another base, yet we could simply dial our home telephone number without a calling card. The phone lines had a specific measure of assigned time each month and found the middle value of out to be around 15 minutes per week for every individual. A similar satellite association provided our web, and we utilized centers to divide interfaces so that everybody could interface from the tasks community in Sharana and all the bunk rooms. As these associations were split between two dozen individuals, the rates were delayed and too delayed to even think about permitting video.

he best technique for correspondence back home was an email, albeit excessively enormous of connections wouldn't send, so I was unable to send such a large number of pictures immediately. The PC that I brought from my home unit was an administration bought strategic framework. Since my PC was government hardware, I could connect it into the unclassified organization the activities place. I utilized the

PC for email, computerized maps, and a radio visit program, and had the option to turn off it and take it back to my B-Hut to watch a film in the evening.

A Wisconsin official counsel financed a web area name, and I made and kept up with the site to assist with imparting our story to relatives. I utilized www.taskforcewisconsin.com to post news refreshes and photographs from the preparation preparing and arrangement, and I utilized some photograph altering abilities and made a logo for our Wisconsin counsel bunch. I posted my photos and a few pictures shared by different individuals from the site all through preparing and sending. Tragically, I encountered trouble keeping up with the website as web accessibility and association speeds were amazingly restricted in Afghanistan.

The most common way of getting mail is very disappointing as it changed relying upon area. In Gardez, a 5-ton truck welcomed the mail on a practically week by week caravan from Camp Phoenix, and there was a little mail center in a B-Hut where you had the option to send bundles. In Sharana, you could depend on counsel escorts through Gardez or utilize the close by

Sharana Provincial Reconstruction Team's mail framework. I wasn't in Bermel sufficiently long to get any mail, yet I might have utilized the Task Force Catamount mail framework on periodic Chinook helicopter flights. Camp Phoenix had customary postal tasks, and I utilized their administration for a couple of enormous boxes and sacks to transport home.

Very barely any Afghan fighters communicated in English, so we required deciphered to interpret our interchanges. At the point when I was in the ordnance organization in Sharana, we had a committed translator, Obie. Beforehand, there were translators for the gathering, and we utilized them when required. In Gardez, when we went to the Afghan Army base for a gathering, the counsel would stop at the translator B-Hut, and a mediator immediately went along. Each of our translators all through the sending were neighborhood nationals chipping away at an agreement with the US military. Obie ended up being an incredible mediator despite the fact that he was somewhat more youthful. I created huge confidence in him, and he had a grip based on ordnance conditions, which is an unmistakable language. I worked with Obie for my span as the battle support counselor, and he was with me for the majority of my missions. Obie was chipping away at getting his Green Card to move to the US, and I kept in touch with him a letter of suggestion before I withdrew. I discovered after my sending that Obie moved to Colorado, and he returned to Afghanistan as a translator for a year and afterward set off for college in the US. I composed a letter of proposal for his lone wolf's and his graduate degree programs. Last I heard, he was completing his graduate degree at Georgetown
University.

NIFORMS AND LAUNDRY

The US Army approved another fight uniform, progressing from the green cover uniform with cleaned dark boots to the dim computerized print uniform with tan calfskin boots. Officers sent to Afghanistan were given the tan cover desert uniform with tan softened cowhide boots. There was vulnerability regarding which uniform we would be given, and a couple of warriors hurried out to buy the new example uniform and boots. I chose to pause and take whatever was issued.

The uniform on the base was a cap and a weapon in yellow status, which means a full magazine embedded and no round of ammo in the chamber. Battle counselors by and large have a M9 9mm gun and a M4 5.56mm rifle. We normally wore the gun in a holster and kept the rifle got in our quarters, and we had the two weapons when we left the base. We wore the Army actual wellness preparing uniform for actual wellness preparing, resting, and personal time. We just had one bunch of regular citizen garments that remained at the lower part of our duffle pack that we could bring while going on our four-day pass or fourteen day leave periods. At the point when we left the base, we were in the full fight pack: gun, rifle, protective cap, body shield with defensively covered plates, emergency treatment unit, and ammo. I connected my ammo magazine pockets to my body protective layer and had seven magazines of rifle ammo and three magazines of gun ammo. I had two discontinuity explosives, a little Garmin GPS, a compass, and a handheld radio on my protection. I utilized my pockets on my uniform to consistently convey my advanced camera, tourniquet, Palm Pilot, couple distinctive little spotlights, and covered cheat cards. I had cheat cards for medevac, call for fire and close air support as these would be the probably going to be utilized. I had a knapsack that contained my night vision goggles, water, snacks, and other fundamental gear.

Overnight stays required a backpack with resting gear, additional garments, and individual cleanliness things. All of this stuff is profound, particularly since our front and back protection plates weighed around six pounds each. As the heavy weapons specialist or on a got off watch, we utilized our freight pockets to store hard confections and different things to give out to the youngsters. The Multi-Band Inter/Intra Team Radio (MBITR) radio is an encoded block size handheld radio that can likewise utilize satellite correspondences. It worked out that my acquisition of an economical Garmin GPS was definitely worth the cost. I utilized my Garmin GPS for the few

times that I expected to give matrix arranges as I didn't have paper guides of our areas.

In Sharana, the climate was somewhat loose around the counselor side of the base. We kept up with prepping norms, however we had a couple of unapproved varieties of Army outfits. For example, everybody had a baseball cap, and the unit coordinations counselor gave me an additional a that had "FD NY" from the 9/11 assaults. We didn't generally wear our uniform coat and frequently moved our sleeves when we wore it, and I didn't generally wear my gun when I was in my actual wellness uniform.

S fighters had night vision goggles that worked by strengthening surrounding light and typically functioned admirably with accessible evening glow however makes a grainy dark and green world. Nonetheless, brilliant lights, like headlights, are likewise escalated, and the night vision goggles would become cleaned out with a radiant green tone. Notwithstanding the grainy dark and greens, night vision goggles don't give any profundity discernment, so making a decision about distance is testing. There is a zeroing in handle on the gadget to change the concentration at various stretches, like optics. I for the most part put away my night vision goggles my rucksack, and my protective cap had a clasp for fast connection. It was trying to utilize the night vision goggles reliably as they had a restricted stock of unique batteries, and they added weight to the protective cap. The Afghan Army didn't have night vision goggles at this time span, so night activities were convoluted. For instance, the Afghan officers would streak the headlights in their pickups to see, yet in doing as such, they would make a waste of time impact with night vision goggles. The impressive larger part of the foe powers didn't have night vision goggles either, so the US fighters enjoyed a distinct benefit. Shockingly, I had practically no night vision goggle preparing or use before my deployment.

concluded that I would bring a couple of Crocs shoes as shower shoes rather than normal flip failures since they would remain on my feet better. I brought a yellow pair along, which made me stand apart strolling to the bathrooms. I utilized the yellow Crocks for some time and changed to red partially through the sending and viewed them as advantageous for strolling on rock or in the snow to the bathrooms. The vast majority of the officers had dark flip lemon, so I was the beneficiary of a ton of peculiar looks.

Shortly in the wake of putting on a uniform, it turned into a sweat-soaked and pungent wreck, and afterward the moon residue would cover everything. It was difficult to get or remain clean. Camp Shelby gave new arrangements of garbs, and I quickly sent one

uniform home so I would have a new uniform after sending. I kept one uniform in the lower part of my duffle sack so I would just utilize it as an extra, and I pivoted two regalia. I didn't have worker for hire support for clothing administrations through my whole arrangement, in the same way as other of the huge bases in Iraq and Afghanistan. The bases had several washers and dryers to help the entire base. I as a rule did clothing one time per week, yet the circumstance would shift because of others sitting tight for the machines. Assuming you didn't investigate the washing, you could track down your wet garments in a heap on top of the washer or the dried garments in a stack on a seat. At the point when I was in Bermel, the dryer was not working, so I needed to dry my garments on a rope clothesline and trust the breeze didn't blow them onto the dusty ground.

YGIENE

One of the most posed inquiries that space travelers get from understudies is the manner by which they go to the restroom in space. Americans take the straightforward object of a latrine for allowed, and it is hard, particularly for more youthful youngsters, to imagine how to direct every day living occasions without the necessities. How could we keep up with our cleanliness and direct our every day living occasions? It relies upon where you were found. Utilizing a washroom consistently required a stroll as there were no on suites or restrooms inside our living regions. The walk found the middle value of around 50 yards, and it very well may be dull and frigid. The more monstrous bases, like Camp Phoenix, had plumbed trailers with a little bank of sinks, six shower slows down, and four latrine slows down. These trailers had heated water, and nearby workers for hire kept up with the tidiness. Medium-sized bases, like Gardez, had a crude substantial structure with sinks, showers, latrines, and clothing with heated water. Little bases, like Bermel, had showers and sinks in a crude substantial construction however had toilets with consume barrels and piss-tubes. Piss-tubes were dispersed all through the base, which was screen covered PVC pipes that were covered in the ground and smelled more awful than the toilets. While I didn't take part, a typical unapproved practice is to keep void Gatorade bottles under your bed to stay away from a late-night walk.

he more modest bases had restricted warm water supply that drew upon the sun warming a dark water tank on the restroom rooftop. We had time limits on showers to guarantee that others had warm water accessible. One day in Sharana, my sergeant counsel was in the shower, and a unit official consultant jabbed his head past the shower shade to advise him to rush... off-kilter! All the shower slows down had some kind of shower shade, generally torn and buildup, and

frequently didn't cover the whole opening, so there would be definitely no real excuse to stick your head into a shower slow down. Away from the base, we expected to burrow a little opening and afterward cover it thereafter. This crouching technique is convoluted with all the stuff's weight and leaves you in a real sense presented to the adversary. I review no less than one escort that needed to stop on the grounds that a battle guide had the runs, and he was crouching on the country road. We would have rather not be assaulted with our jeans down!

I utilized an electric razor for shaving and had a little, battery-worked shaver to take in my short-term sack during transient status or on the lookout. I additionally had a Mach 3 razor and shaving cream, however I didn't utilize it frequently as running, high temp water was restricted. The more monstrous bases had a barbershop for hair styles. Since I was at a more modest base, I didn't get the chance to visit the hair stylist except if I went through the more broad base. I bought a hair trimmer and trim my hair with the number two-watch. Two or three different guides had hair trimmers as well and given hair styles, yet I felt remorseful asking them when I could do it myself.

WATER

The water in the sinks on the bases was undependable to drink, so all water burned-through was from plastic jugs. Assuming you were going on a got off watch, it was for the most part better to fill a CamelBak hydration framework with the plastic water bottles. The CamelBak's drinking tube was near the head for accommodation, however I observed the CamelBak testing to spotless and an agony to fill. It was simpler to utilize plastic water bottles around the base or in the firearm trucks. Rather than utilizing the CamelBak on watches, I would guarantee that I had a few water bottles in my rucksack. We generally had water cases in the weapon truck and by our bunks, and we expected to bring a water jug to the bathroom to clean our teeth. I would become extremely worn out on drinking plain water. More often than not, the water bottles were not refrigerated, and we devoured them at room temperature. Assuming we put away water bottles in the weapon truck, they would regularly be hot. The water was somewhat better in case you had some Crystal Light or other character bundles to add. I don't think I at any point saw ice for the whole organization. The vast majority of the bases had some refrigeration, so there was a restricted inventory of cold water bottles. There was by and large Gatorade accessible alongside some caffeinated drinks. In the main portion of the sending, Red Bull was accessible in certain areas, however constantly half, RipIts supplanted the Red Bulls. On the subject of beverages, liquor was restricted by all US military

individuals, however a few nearby bases had Bitburger non-hard brew available.

FOOD

Eating on an Air Force base is in every case better compared to an Army base, and the best feasting office I ate at was in Qatar. Project workers arranged suppers in Camp Phoenix, and Gardez resembled an inferior quality school home corridor. The menu looked more invigorating than how it tasted, particularly the week after week shrimp and steak suppers. I was energized toward the start of the sending when I discovered that we would have steak and crab legs, yet all the same wound up painfully disillusioned. After I cut the grizzly fat off, I was left with a few chomps of all around good done chewy meat. The crab legs had adaptable, rubbery shells that our plastic blade couldn't cut, and in case you figured out how to detach the shell, all that remained was a little overcooked nibbles swimming in a water and margarine sauce. Camp Phoenix and Gardez had a little self-service counter and Jell-O, and I would extraordinarily see the value in the new vegetables toward the finish of the deployment.

Bermel had a few Task Force Catamount cooks that for the most part served the pre-arranged dinners, however they energized it up, and their suppers were superior to the project workers at the more huge bases, and they did it with less assets. The best part was that they had frozen yogurt accessible and steady coffee.

Sharana didn't have a US eating office or any food administration faculty. Battle consultants would need to escort to Sharana Provincial Reconstruction Team sometimes to get food supplies, dry products, and semi-arranged dinners. The semi-arranged supper is a feast pack to take care of a unit and regularly comes in huge plastic-type sacks that you could hotness and serve, bigger and like the renowned Meal Ready to Eat (MREs). The US groups' arrangement was to alternate to prepare a supper feast, and everybody was all alone for breakfast and lunch. I elected to prepare supper all the more regularly, as I wasn't completely engaged.

n the initial fourteen days, I prepared supper five evenings. Preparing supper was a tedious interaction. We didn't have an oven or broiler, and our cooler space was restricted. The storage space had a little microwave and a hot plate; in any case, it would trip the electrical switch assuming that you turned both on simultaneously. We utilized the outside barbecue as our oven to prepare supper. The fuel supply for the outside barbecue was a square of super hardwood. Since we didn't have fuel to light a normal fire, we splashed the hardwood lumps in diesel fuel for two hours. Then, at that point, we would light the splashed hardwood and consume it for close to 60 minutes to get all the diesel out. We could cook with our restricted pots and container and get all that set up to serve at 6:00 pm.

I cooked spaghetti and meatballs, pan sear, greasy steaks a few times, and burgers. Steaks were by a long shot the most straightforward to get ready, and that was the default dinner for some others, yet in no way, shape or form were they quality meats. Generally, we began splashing the hardwood around 2:00 pm and wrapped tidying up the pots and skillet by 7:00 pm. We didn't have a full supplement of kitchen apparatuses and utensils and would need to be innovative in planning. We didn't have a colander, so when I made spaghetti noodles in an immense pot, I utilized the cover and painstakingly adjusted the hot pot to deplete the water. Breakfast most days was a Pop-Tart, and lunch was for the most part Ramen noodles. I every so often had Ramen or popcorn for supper in the event that somebody consumed the steaks or couldn't prepare supper.

VEHICLES

Weapon truck – M114A2, Up-Armored High Mobility Multipurpose Wheeled Vehicle (HMMWV). This vehicle has a shield bundle that can give assurance against an AK-47 or gunnery parts. There are four awkward seats and a spot on the back console that an officer can bear operating the weighty weapon. An assortment of weapons can join in the turret, including medium assault rifles, substantial assault rifles, and programmed projectile launchers.

Our firearm trucks were seven and a half-ton skewed back reinforced vehicles with an underpowered super diesel motor. The weapon turret had a short protective layer plate around the incubate opening on the rooftop, and there was a reinforcement safeguard that everybody called a chicken safeguard. The weapon truck had a radiator for winter and a climate control system for summer, yet I don't remember a period that the bring forth on the turret was shut to make either successful. In the warm months, the heavy armament specialist could partake in the dusty breeze, and the driver could partake in some problematic cooling. In the chilly months, the heavy armament specialist would freeze, however the driver would get a little warm air. Driving the firearm truck was somewhat precarious as the windows were unbeatable and stayed shut and brought about negligible perspectives. The driver would need to depend on input from the heavy armament specialist for perception, particularly towards the back. The vast majority of the weapon trucks had an inner headset framework for the heavy armament specialist, driver, and traveler to convey as the firearm truck was very uproarious with its turbodiesel motor operating.

Other US military units had different sorts of vehicles. The most well-known vehicle other than the weapon truck was a material covered five-ton freight truck. These six-wheeled trucks had a covering assurance bundle on the taxi and

automatic weapon mount. I needed to ride toward the rear of a freight truck on one of the legs of my movements to Bagram for my four-day pass in December. The course between Camp Phoenix and Bagram was moderately protected, yet we needed to remain low to the floor of the freight bed, and there was no insurance. Firearm trucks would give an escort to the guard. It was so cold and breezy, so I folded my camping cot over me to keep warm.

The other US military vehicle that I got a kick out of the chance to see was the course leeway trucks. Sadly, there was a shortage and were for the most part utilized for bigger guards. I just review two caravans with the course freedom bundle. A course leeway bundle normally comprised of adjusted street grader that could check for side of the road bombs and an angular heavily clad truck to convey the specialist support troopers. The street conditions forestalled most other military trucks as they would be excessively weighty or excessively huge to drive.

In 2006, there was just a single fundamental cleared interstate, the Ring Road, which was a huge circle around the center of the country. Kabul and a couple of other bigger urban areas had central avenues cleared with pot-holed concrete. The vast majority of the other principle streets were semi-worked on compacted country roads, and any vehicles or trucks would create a little residue storm. As you were further from the urban communities, the roads deteriorated to unchanged country roads and dry waterway beds. There were just a modest bunch of escorts that voyaged quicker than 20 miles each hour During every one of my watches and the vast majority of my guards, we were unable to go quicker than 20 miles each hour as the streets had an excessive number of potholes, grooves, and craters.

Most of the Afghan vehicles and trucks were more established and messy varieties of a Toyota Corolla or little Toyota pickups. There were a great deal of cruisers and enormous jingle trucks for pulling wood and supplies. A jingle truck is an enormous Afghan freight truck utilized like semi-trucks inside the US. Since the street conditions are so poor inside the country, semi-trucks can't cross the streets. A jingle truck is like an enormous box U-Haul truck without a rooftop, and Afghans will normally paint the trucks with splendid shadings and connect ringers and chains for the truck to make jingle commotions while driving the harsh streets. US powers would infrequently contract jingle trucks to ship fuel or delivery containers.

WEAPONS

Heavy assault rifle – M2 Browning Machine Gun, .50 type. This 83-pound short force weapon can precisely shoot a shot with regards to the size of a thumb 2,000 yards. This automatic rifle can start up to 850 rounds each moment with a greatest scope of 8,100 yards, and can rapidly annihilate a motor square on a vehicle. This weighty assault rifle is extremely scary yet additionally confounded. The weighty barrel is a different part, however they can't be exchanged with other automatic weapons. When the heavy armament specialist screws the coordinated with barrel into the automatic rifle, he then, at that point, utilizes an uncommon instrument to gauge the headspace between the barrel and weapon to guarantee the circumstance will consider constant fire.

Medium assault rifle – M240B Machine Gun, 7.62mm. The 27 pound, open bolt automatic weapon can precisely shoot a slug 875 yards. This automatic weapon can start up to 600 rounds each moment with a most extreme scope of 4,000 yards. The medium automatic weapon is flexible and can be utilized on a bipod, firearm truck, or helicopter.

Rifle – M4A2 5.56mm supplanted the famous M16 rifle. Significant enhancements incorporated a folding stock and a rail connection framework rather than standard handguards around the barrel. The folding stock was intended to have better control in restricted spaces, similar to room clearing, yet was a distinct benefit for more modest height troopers such as myself. There were various connections for the rail framework; the military gave a few, and warriors could purchase others. The military furnished me with a red spot optic sight, Surefire electric lamp, and an infrared laser pointer. Many officers purchased unique handgrips and bipods. The standard magazine held 30 rounds, and we conveyed no less than seven magazines on our body armor.

Pistol – M9 Beretta gun is expected to be a reinforcement weapon. Most battle counsels had a rifle and a gun, yet everybody had a prerequisite to convey no less than one weapon, so the gun was a lot more straightforward to haul around the base. The 9mm gun has a viable short-range and was expected to progress from a rifle failure to fire to tight situation shooting rapidly. The standard magazine held ten rounds, and we conveyed three extra magazines on our body armor.

AFGHAN CULTURE

Afghanistan is one of the most monetarily immature underdeveloped nations on the planet. Significant commodities are nuts and opium, and Afghanistan has a critical stockpile of lapis lazuli, an uncommon dazzling blue stone. Monetary guide and the commonplace reproduction groups buckled down, working on country roads and making more cleared streets. Little mud homes and hand-worked fields spotted the open country. Man centric families stayed extremely close and didn't notice kid work laws as it was pervasive to see small kids working around the home and fields.

ver 95% of the Afghan public are Muslim and follow various qualities and morals than most Americans. Perhaps the most clear difference was the different brings to supplication over the amplifiers for the duration of the day and the Muslim sacred day was Friday. There wasn't preparing booked on Fridays nor numerous missions, so the counsels utilized Fridays as our low functional beat days to clean the firearm trucks and weapons, watch films, or do clothing. I learned not to sit with your heels pointing at somebody, shake with just the right hand, and the standard hello and answer, "Salaam-Alaikum and Alaikum-Salaam" which means "Harmony be unto you" and "unto your peace."

e heard bits of hearsay and jokes about "man love Thursdays" and "ladies are for multiplication and young men are for diversion." I don't have any proof of the reality of these tales, yet when the mediators prescribe not going to the Afghan Army side on Thursday nights, I will generally trust the narratives. I never went to the Afghan Army side on a Thursday night. It was additionally omnipresent for male Afghan Army troopers to clasp hands, which shows their companionship and trust. I saw a couple of guides clasping hands with their Afghan Army warriors, however I didn't take part in this custom.

e heard a great deal about debasement and how it was very nearly an assumption in their way of life. The extortion was far reaching, from an Afghan Police designated spot requesting pay-offs to Afghan Army pioneers taking additional address and project workers checking costs for rock. We heard a typical grievance from the Afghan Army fighters that they were not paid or didn't accept their full installment amount.

The Afghans have powerful connections to family and clans and don't frequently perceive the public authority and regularly have quarrels among clans going on for ages. With the various loyalties, defilement, and debates, you had no clue about what the Afghan Army or local people's actual expectations were.

Our military is exceptionally effective and has time principles, destinations, and purposes. Numerous Afghans had the overall disposition of "Inshallah," signifying "in the event that God wills it." Most Afghans don't have tickers or schedules, and many don't have a clue about their birthday or age. Some Afghan Army utilized "Inshalla" when shooting their AK-47s, accepting they can point the weapon the overall way; in the event that God wills it, the projectile will descend upon the adversary. It was unquestionably baffling attempting to pass on the significance of time, arranging, and in reverse planning.

INTO THE STAN

"Some of the time you end up in the center of no place, and in some cases in no place you find yourself."

Anonymous

The day of our departure from Camp Shelby was also the day we were supposed to start taking doxycycline, a daily anti-malaria medication. Wake up time was 3:00 am, and we hurried to lead individual cleanliness and get together our final things to stack into the truck. I took my drug portion with a taste of water when I woke up so I could pack.
Within a brief time, I was overwhelmed with sickness and was dry hurling in the bathroom as opposed to stacking the truck — what an extraordinary method for beginning the flight day. Example learned – have drug with food. That day was a ton of pick up the pace and pause, with stacking the truck with things, transport ride to the air terminal, lounging around the holder for quite a long time, lastly stacking into a contracted business aircraft. With the size of the airplane and the quantity of us flying, I had three seats to myself and partook in the window view.

We showed up at Manas Air Force Base in Kyrgyzstan right away before 12 PM on February 24th, beginning our time limit of 365 days in theater. We remained as homeless people in lofts in extremely jam-packed tents with nothing to accomplish for a couple of days. In case you were unfortunate to be in the top bunk, you had the wind current, light, and top of the tent inside a few inches. Being 5'6" tall and 150 pounds, I was unfortunate. Since this was an Air Force base, the suppers at the eating office were heavenly as everything is better in the Air Force.

Our Wisconsin guide group wound up on the initial gigantic fly freight plane turn into Kabul International Airport on February 27th. The C-17 fly freight plane was striking. Like all tactical airplane, we needed to wear ear security because of the clamor levels. It was stunning how quick and far this plane can fly conveying such a lot of freight. This plane was intended to convey 100 airborne troopers with their gear more than 6,000 miles however can convey however much an Abrams tank. Being inside caused me to feel little. Despite the fact that this was a gigantic airplane, it could take-off rapidly, land on short runways, and has the abilities of making a few G-powers during flying moves. Flying corps work force palletized our sacks and sacks, and we conveyed our defensive stuff and void weapons. Part of the way through the flight, the pilot wound down the lights and educated everybody to put on their head protectors as we were over an antagonistic country. I put on my head protector and was pondering the conceivable forthcoming threats. After we landed, we were each given a fractional magazine for our guns, and we boarded a transport with drapes on the windows. A transport took us to Camp Phoenix, close to the east finish of Kabul. I was a little befuddled with regards to the genuine threats as we needed to put our head protectors on during the flight, and presently, we had a transport ride in Kabul city with curtains covering the windows.

Once all the counselor groups from Camp Shelby showed up at Camp Phoenix, we started briefings and preparing. One of the security briefings clarified how much feces was noticeable all around from the open sewage … it will be an extraordinary year! We had a short class on the strategic satellite radio, which was helpful as we could go through the radio and set the compact satellite recieving wire. We had a brief period for drivers preparing and had the option to drive the up-reinforced Humvee, alluded to as firearm trucks, not too far off from Camp Phoenix and encountered some insane traffic in Kabul. There were no settled standards of the street for Afghan drivers and just had two or three overall rules. The roads that we drove on were two pieces of asphalt that mixed into the hard pack soil among the outdoors shops. For the most part, drivers drove on the right-hand side of the cleared strip, and there were no street markings, so everybody went their own speed, attempting to keep away from one another and the various potholes.

During our couple of days in Camp Phoenix, a few other remarkable occasions happened. To start with, I encountered my first seismic tremor. A few of us were unwinding in the transient B-Hut and felt an unexpected thundering. I had my earphones in my ears while watching a film and didn't quickly have a clue what was occurring. One sergeant counsel shouted that it should be approaching discharge and snatched his gun and ran out the secondary passage without his protective cap or body reinforcement. One more sergeant consultant, who was from California, immediately said it was a quake. I didn't have the foggiest idea what the sergeant counselor planned to do with his gun against approaching mortar discharge. Second, President George W. Hedge had a visit to Kabul. I didn't be familiar with his visit on March first, and I saw a lot of assault helicopters zooming around, which appeared to be somewhat uncommon. I discovered the following day that President Bush and the First Lady, Barbara Bush, were in Kabul and Bagram Air Force Base for an astonishment visit.

The US order structure was a perplexing wire chart with a few diverse order connections. A three-star general, Lieutenant General Karl Eikenberry, directed the Combined Forces Command – Afghanistan. It was settled in Bagram and composed with the International Security Assistance Force (ISAF), the consulates and other conciliatory missions. Under Combined Forces Command – Afghanistan was the base camp of the tenth Mountain Division and was instructed by a two-star general, Major General Benjamin Freakly. The tenth Mountain Division was answerable for the essential counterinsurgency tasks, overcoming foe powers, and controlling the Provincial Reconstruction Teams that gave common undertakings and designer backing to improve the nearby framework. The other component under Combined Forces Command – Afghanistan was Task Force Phoenix. Their central goal was to prepare the Afghan Army and Afghan Police to lead supported, autonomous counterinsurgency tasks in Afghanistan. A one-star general told Task Force Phoenix, Brigadier General John Perryman, and comprised of all the counselor groups from different states and nations (Canada, Romania, France, and others). The tenth Mountain Division units that I upheld were: second Battalion 87th Infantry, tenth Mountain Division, alluded to as Task Force Catamount and fourth Battalion 25th Field Artillery, tenth Mountain Division, alluded to as Task Force Wolfpack.

The battle consultant was not an officer, so we were unable to coordinate developments or missions of the Afghan Army units. We had a necessity to be with the Afghan Army for direction and mix of the International Security Assistance Force and tenth Mountain Division tasks. Battle consultant channels followed a portion of the missions, and the tenth Mountain Division followed others. More often than not, it seemed like we had many supervisors, yet we were unable to guide anybody. This namelessness likewise left the battle counselor scrambling for assets, including air and cannons support, clinical help, and means. Numerous ordinary officers did not know what a battle counsel was for sure our main goal was. Things are considerably more confounded by adding different countries, Special Operations Forces, other government offices, non-government offices, and project workers. During activation preparing, we got guidance on leading study hall preparing and instructing through a mediator. I would come to learn over the course of the following year that a battle counsel wasn't teaching in the classroom.

Combat guides played three primary parts: self-sustainment, battle enhancers, and hands on guidance. We needed to generally uphold ourselves by doing our clothing, keeping up with our weapons and vehicles, and a huge load of different obligations and obligations. A battle counsel is an essential connection for air, field cannons, and medevac support on Afghan Army missions and the basic connection between International Security Assistance Force and the Afghan Army. During my whole organization as a battle counsel, I was distinctly in a study hall setting once. The vast majority of my mentorship happened as hands on preparing on battle watches and sitting in certain gatherings. Most missions, I would interface up with the Afghan Army official in-control and ensured he actually look at his warriors and was prepared. Notwithstanding, the battle consultant directed a large portion of the Afghan Army missions.

obbit is military vernacular for a warrior who scarcely, if at any time, leaves "the wire" or edge of the base. Organization as a Fobbit is viewed as protected from risk and can make an every day showing and appreciate somewhat fair everyday environments and base conveniences. A Fobbit sending can be exceptionally everyday and slow personal time and have zero involvement in the neighborhood culture. There is enmity between a Fobbit and the warfighter. The warfighter invests energy outside of the wire leading missions. While presented to huge risks, the warfighter will have significantly more different encounters. Both warfighters and Fobbits are needed as there is a requirement for a very long time and occupations. Counsels could commonly fit inside two classifications: unit and higher counselors inside the Fobbit domain and brigade and friends consultants inside the warfighter domain. I appreciated visiting the huge bases to utilize a portion of the conveniences, however wouldn't have any desire to be a Fobbit there for a year.

Our Wisconsin counsel group and the other eight consultant groups from Camp Shelby were split between the five Afghan Army corps a couple of days subsequent to showing up at Camp Phoenix. Generally 50% of our Wisconsin counselor group was split to 205th Afghan Army Corps in

Kandahar Air Force Base in the south, and the other gathering was split to 203rd Afghan Army Corps in Gardez in the east. 203rd Afghan Army Corps has liability regarding Paktia,

Paktika, Ghazni, and Khowst territories, a region most popular for Operation Anaconda in March 2002 with the Battle of Takur Ghar.

There are five Afghan Army corps regions in Afghanistan, assigned as 201st Afghan Army Corps around Kabul, 203rd Afghan Army Corps in the east, 205th Afghan Army Corps in the south, 207th Afghan Army Corps in the west, and 209th Afghan Army Corps in the north. 203rd Afghan Army Corps had two detachments, and each unit had five contingents: three infantry, one battle backing, and one help support. An infantry brigade has four infantry organizations and a central command organization. The battle support brigade comprised of surveillance, architect, big guns, and base camp organizations. The help support regiment has upkeep, transportation, clinical, sign, and central command organizations.

A company is a military unit consisting of 80 – 150 personnel and organized into several platoons. A Captain commands a company, and has the same functional mission and is subordinate to a battalion. A battalion is a military unit consisting of three to seven companies, or 300 – 800 soldiers. The infantry is most associated with battalions; however, there are other functional battalions, such as artillery, military police, combat support, and others. Lieutenant Colonels usually command battalions and are subordinate to a brigade. A brigade is a military unit consisting of three to six battalions with 1,000 to 5,000 soldiers. A Colonel commands a brigade and is subordinate to a division or corps.

There are two main groups of soldiers within the military, enlisted and officer. The enlisted rank is below a commissioned officer and includes sergeants and soldiers that perform jobs specific to their occupations specialty and comprises approximately 80% of the military. The ranks progress from Private to Command Sergeant Major. An officer is a rank in a position of authority and are considered commanding officers under presidential authority. Officers receive their commission from the President upon completion of a variety of programs, such as West Point Military Academy or ROTC. Officers are trained in functional areas but are managers and commanders of programs and personnel. The ranks progress from Second Lieutenant to General.

Our convoy arrived in Gardez after dark, and the base was under blackout conditions, so it was tough to see anything or see anyone. Upon arrival, we found out that we were splitting up again between two brigades. Our smaller group went to the second brigade operations center and found out we were

splitting again among the five Afghan battalions. My first assignment was a brigade signal officer advisor and assisting the brigade personnel officer with Afghan Army pay operations. The new brigade logistics officer advisor, a sergeant advisor, and I had to spend the first few nights in the transient tent and could move to the empty B-Hut once the limited gym equipment was moved out about a week later. Ideally, a brigade advisor team would consist of 16 officers and sergeants, providing mentorship for Afghan Army leaders, personnel, operations, logistics, signal, and medical operations. A battalion advisor team would ideally consist of 16 officers and sergeants, with eight staff in the headquarters and an officer and a sergeant at each company. With limited manpower creating vacancies, rotations, and personnel taking leave, it was prevalent to operate at 50-75% of the authorized strength.

he first four days were dull, and I attempted to figure out where everything was located and meeting different people, both US and Afghan. A sergeant advisor and I cleaned the heavy machine gun, medium machine gun, and the automatic grenade launcher. I was going to be the gunner the next day on the automatic grenade launcher. The sergeant advisor provided excellent instruction on firing, assembly, and cleaning the automatic grenade launcher as the mobilization station did not provide training on this weapon. As I was to learn, the brigade advisor team doesn't conduct combat patrol missions. It will occasionally perform a ground assault convoy to Camp Phoenix for Afghani currency and pick up the mail. A ground assault convoy refers to moving vehicles from one base to another, while a mounted patrol is to conduct a specific mission.

This mission was a little different as it was a convoy to the base in Sharana to survey the base. As a part of the spring re-stationing plan, the Afghan Army brigade headquarters and their advisors would be moving from Gardez to Sharana. The Afghan Army base and the Afghan district governor's complex, co-located on the outskirts of Sharana, and was approximately five miles northwest of the Sharana Provincial Reconstruction Team. The actual name of the base wasn't official, and we referred to it in several ways and eventually was referred to as Sharana, but would often have to clarify it as the Afghan Army Sharana base. The route to base was going through the city of Gardez and taking a dirt road for almost two hours.

The distance was only about 40 miles, but the dirt road was so bad that we often drove slower than 12 miles per hour. Moreover, the dust was extreme.

The dust isn't a problem if you are in the lead vehicle. I had on my goggles

and used a dew rag to cover my mouth and nose and ended up covered in a dust layer. Upon return to Gardez, the automatic grenade launcher was so dust-covered that I am not sure if it would fire. Sharana was in pretty bad condition, and the Afghan Army battalion and their advisors were working with the best they had. We left a sergeant there with funding to improve the conditions by adding protection walls, creating an outdoor fire pit kitchen area, and adding toilets in the latrine building.

The brigade team leader gave me the nickname "Scooter" as my last name was difficult to pronounce. For the first month in Gardez, life and operations tempo was pretty mundane and seemed pretty similar to a regular job and not a combat deployment. A typical day would be to wake up, eat breakfast, go to the operations center, take a break for lunch, back to the operations center, eat dinner, shower, and watch a movie. Typically, I worked on setting up a computer program with digital maps, establishing connections that allowed chat on the computers using the radios instead of the internet, maintaining the Blue Force Tracker in the vehicles, and loading radios with the weekly communications security. The Blue Force Tracker is a touch-screen computer system in the front passenger seat, connected via satellite to other Blue Force Trackers. It would display a digital map with icons and could send electronic messages. The two significant issues with the Blue Force Tracker are that not all vehicles had them installed. Many missions only had two combat advisors as a driver and gunner, so there wasn't an operator for the Blue Force Tracker. Our operations center B-Hut had a few office spaces and a small conference area in the middle where I set up a small work area. We used the conference area for team meetings, cleaning weapons, and general conversations, which resulted in no privacy.

I wasn't a direct mentor but occasionally went to the Afghan Army side of the camp with the brigade personnel officer advisor for Afghan Army pay operations and to meet with the Afghan Army brigade communications team. During this time in the war, designated US personnel would be responsible for the Afghan Army soldiers' accountability and paying them in Afghani every month.

I was in a few meetings with Afghan Army officers and hesitantly accepted chai tea. The Afghan Army didn't have sanitation standards and never washed the teacups. The teacups looked like they had a layer of slime on them as the Afghans only rinsed them, and I learned to drink from above the handle of the cup, which was likely the cleanest area. I also toured the

Afghan Army dining facility, which made my stomach turn with the cooking conditions. The kitchen area was covered in dense smoke from the wood fires, and the entire area was covered in dirt and soot. Metal buckets were overfilling with some kind of raw, fatty meat joints and stacks of naan bread on the tables.

On March 18th, we had a three-day convoy to Bagram Air Force base, through Camp Phoenix, to get briefed on the changes to the Afghan Army pay operations and pick up some vehicle parts from depot maintenance. I operated the heavy machine gun for the uneventful convoy. On March 22nd, I was tasked to go on a combat patrol with an infantry company combat advisor to establish traffic control checkpoints. I was the medium machine gunner, and we followed the Afghan Army soldiers in their tan Ford Ranger pickups, to what seemed like the middle of nowhere. There was an intersection of two dirt roads in a broad valley, and our gun truck provided overwatch for the checkpoint. I think there were only a few civilian vehicles that came to the checkpoint all morning. After our checkpoint mission, we drove to a nearby small village. We dismounted the vehicles and walked into the village, and the combat advisors spoke with a teacher who understood some English. A couple of others and I handed out some candy and school supplies that we brought along. Afterward, we went back to our vehicles and returned to base. It was pretty uneventful for my first combat patrol.

Later that night, an explosion sounded off in the distance, and people started yelling "incoming." The brigade logistics officer advisor, the sergeant advisor, and I quickly put on our body armor and helmet and went into the nearby bunker, an open concrete tube covered with sandbags. This attack was only one rocket that fell beyond the perimeter. Somebody eventually came by and asking for names for accountability, and they gave the all-clear after 30 minutes. Leadership told me that rockets' threat was low as the enemy did not have an effective way to aim the rocket. The enemy usually propped the rockets up with rocks or a makeshift stand and used the Kentucky windage to point in the general direction. Since the local event did not have an ample supply of rockets and did not have sophisticated aiming devices, any rocket attacks on our base would be infrequent and ineffective.

On select days, local Afghans set up a bazaar in the Provincial Reconstruction Team in Gardez, a short convoy outside of Gardez. A bazaar is similar to a flea or farmers market, where local vendors would set up a temporary market monitored by the base. The Afghans would have tarps and tents set up to sell black-market movies, knock off watches, gems and jewelry, rugs, fancy wood boxes, and some other items. Having the skills for negotiations and using an interpreter is handy as the prices were always flexible and changing. Most of the bases had the occasional bazaar, and I shopped at them in Bagram, Camp Phoenix, Gardez Provincial Reconstruction Team, and Orgun-E and bought a few movies and trinkets. I did buy four of the fancy wood jewelry boxes that I would give my wife and to my nieces for Christmas. Shipping the boxes and other items home proved to be a whole separate frustrating process.

bout one month after being assigned as the signal officer, the brigade team leader asked me how I felt about becoming a team chief on the Romanian advisor battalion team. Four days later, he told me that I would be reassigned to the Afghan Army 1st Infantry Battalion on April 7th as the battalion team leader. The day before my reassignment, the brigade advisor team took a short patrol into Gardez to visit the fortress and the disarmament, demobilization, and reintegration site. I was awestruck by the size of the fortress. I believe the 3rd Corps of the former Afghan Army used the massive fort. The disarmament, demobilization, and reintegration site were located in the northern part of Gardez and was the boneyard for all the tanks, trucks, equipment, and weapons from the Russian invasion. The equipment was all non-operational as it was missing engines and principal components. I found it very interesting to see the actual Russian weapons that I spent a lot of time memorizing on flashcards in the Field Artillery Officer Basic Course in 1998. Afterward, our interpreters bought us lunch from a local vendor, and I enjoyed my first real Afghan meal with rice and kabobs made with naan, lamb, onion, and cilantro.

VAMPIRES

"The strength of the vampire is that people will not believe in him." – Garrett Hill

The Afghan Army 1st Battalion combat advisor team structure was unique. On the tracking spreadsheet, there was one US officer position mentoring the Afghan Army battalion personnel officer and one US sergeant mentor in the headquarters company. The rest of the advisor team was 21 Romanian officers and sergeants, led by a Romanian Major. Romania deployed its soldiers with only an AK-47 rifle; therefore, Task Force Phoenix had to supply all the equipment. For accountability purposes, there was a requirement for a US officer to be assigned with the Romanians to handle funding and hand receipt all the equipment, vehicles, and heavy weapons. For all practical purposes, I was the senior advisor on the team as I attended the brigade meetings and mentored the Afghan Army battalion commander and executive officer. Gross, a new sergeant, assigned to the battalion team, became the paying agent, interpreter manager, and mentored the senior Afghan Army sergeants. We had a gun truck with a heavy machine gun and a gun truck with a medium machine gun for the Romanian advisor. We were also responsible for six pickups for the remaining Romanian soldiers, along with radios and some other equipment. A couple of weeks later, a new officer advisor assumed the responsibilities for logistics officer and hand receipts. ur advisor team radio call sign was "vampire," and Gross and I made a stencil of a vampire bat to put on the doors of our gun trucks.

The Afghan Army battalion had a weekly responsibility to provide a checkpoint on Terra Pass, about a 30-minute drive into the mountains, to provide security for the Afghan Army corps leadership to travel home to Kabul on Thursdays and return on Saturdays. Typically, about a dozen Afghan Army soldiers in pickups and a few advisors, usually the Romanians, would conduct this operation for a half day. Gross and I went a couple of times in the gun truck, and it seemed to waste half of a day. The Afghan Army officers would have a couple of Afghan Army soldiers climb the nearby mountains, and a few Afghan Army soldiers would stand by their pickups. The combat advisors stayed by the Afghan Army pickup. The Afghan Army wasn't allowed to stop the vehicles passing by, so everyone sat around for several hours, watching the vehicles drive by and providing a presence.

On April 26th and 27th, the Afghan Army battalion was tasked to provide long-duration dismounted patrols to increase the Gardez security presence. Gross and I took about a dozen Afghan Army soldiers on two very long foot patrols, walking around the city. We patrolled eight miles the first day and six miles the second day. I was sore, sweaty, and sunburned. I was not physically prepared to conduct a long foot patrol as I was an artillery officer and moved by vehicles. These foot patrols made me dig down deep to keep going as I didn't want to appear weak in front of the Afghan Army soldiers, even though I had on my complete gear and the Afghan soldiers had a helmet and AK-47.

We participated with the "hearts and minds" campaign by handing out balloons and candy to the local children. Otherwise, the patrols were uneventful.

One of my primary focus areas was to ensure a smooth transition of Romanian advisors as the entire Romanian team was leaving, and a new team would be arriving. I worked with the brigade team leader for a transfer of authority ceremony and presented each soldier with a certificate. Most of our efforts were developing a training plan for the incoming Romanian advisors for our vehicles, weapons, and radios, as this would be all new equipment for them. Gross was the primary instructor, and I assisted and taught a couple of classes. The Romanian advisors received training on Blue Force Tracker, communications, close air support, medevac requests, medium machine gun, and gun truck familiarization over nine days and included firing on the range. The new Romanian team seemed to have a better attitude than the previous group and took the training well. Training the Romanian team is how I envisioned my deployment when I was first notified of the mission. We had small group classes, demonstrations, and practices.

I was busier with team chief responsibilities as opposed to my previous assignment as a signal officer. The Romanians were notorious for being difficult to work with as they used minimal efforts and had language barriers. Only two or three of the Romanians knew English, and the rest knew Romanian and some Russian. The language barriers are challenging as the Afghan Army soldiers spoke different dialects, our interpreters spoke English and some Afghan dialects, and the Romanians spoke Romanian, Russian and some English. I had to use a Romanian officer as a translator to talk to the Romanian Major as he only knew Romanian. The Romanian soldiers were not subject to alcohol restrictions to have beer and alcohol in their B-Huts. I was in charge of the team, but I did not have any authority over the Romanians and most often seemed like dreaded babysitting duty.

hortly after the Romanians completed their training, I focused heavily on the spring re-stationing plan. Gardez contained most of the Afghan Army brigade, and the idea was to relocate around the area to other bases. The Afghan Army battalion was to transfer to Bermel and the border control point in Shkin to replace the unit there who would relocate to Gardez for lower operational tempo. Many considered Bermel and Shkin to be one of the most hostile areas in Afghanistan at the time. The Afghan Army battalion there had been conducting operations in the area for a while with their combat advisors of US Marine Corps (Marines) from 2nd Battalion 3rd Marine Regiment. The border control point was an Afghan Army-operated site, with only a couple of structures for barracks. A company of Afghan Army would occupy on a monthly rotation with the rest of the battalion in Bermel.

Directly across the 100-yard border were a Pakistan checkpoint and an observation bunker on the top of the adjacent hill, which could observe the entire area. On top of one of the buildings in Pakistan was the Taliban flag, which makes you wonder Pakistan's alliance status. Outside nations only recognized this border as the locals all referred to this 7,200 square miles area of Afghanistan and Pakistan as Waziristan and tribes controlled the area. A few Marine Combat Advisors resided at Shkin, nestled in the mountains about six miles from the border control point. Most of the other residents at Shkin were personnel from Special Forces and other government agencies. Task Force Wolfpack had a small section assigned to Shkin to provide artillery support with their 105mm howitzer.

n April 19th, I went on a Blackhawk helicopter flight for leader visits to Bermel and Lwara. A Blackhawk helicopter, UH-60 Sikorsky aircraft, is a four-blade, twin-engine, medium-lift helicopter designed to carry 11 equipped troops. This helicopter has a range of 370 miles at 170 miles per hour, and usually has medium machine guns mounted on the side door. This visit allowed me to meet the combat advisors that we would be replacing and check out the base. We first flew to Lwara, and I saw a fellow Wisconsin officer advisor, who was getting ready for a mission. I tagged along on the base visit to see their operations center and their small base. Lwara sat in the mountains with the full surrounding of mountains. An advisor explained that the Afghan Army soldiers used goats to move supplies up the mountain to the observation points. I was able to see how the Afghans made naan bread and why it was called "foot bread." The Afghan Army had two local bakers making fresh naan daily in a small kitchen building. It wasn't much of a kitchen as it was the size of a small office and had a hole in the middle of the dirty plywood floor that was the oven. One man was making the dough, and one man would stretch it out using his foot and then slap it against the inside of the oven. Even though the Afghan man made it with his foot, the naan tasted great.

Our gathering then, at that point, traveled to Bermel, and the Marine insight official counsel directed me around the base, both on the US and Afghan Army sides. We didn't get to visit Shkin or the line control point, as Shkin was toward the south, and the line control point was toward the southeast. I took many pictures on our short visit and acquired resources for coordination.

On May tenth, at around 11:30 pm in Gardez, I was again stirred by a blast's sound. There were yells outside the B-Hut demonstrating approaching rocket fire. I promptly put on my defensive gear and answered to our activities community. At the activities community, I met Gross, and we each got a handheld radio. Gross began taking responsibility of the Romanian work force as they were just in the country for a couple of days, and this was their first backhanded assault. I answered to the unit tasks focus to check in with the detachment group pioneer. Simultaneously, we dispatched two Romanians to the Afghan Army region to take responsibility. Following a couple of moments, we represented every Romanian officer, aside from one was absent. I kept on remaining in the detachment activities focus to screen the circumstance. Simultaneously, Gross and a few senior Romanian counselors endeavored to search for the missing Romanian, nicknamed "Frozen yogurt." After a brief time, somebody observed the Romanian official stowing away under a truck, and the two Romanians returned from the contingent with the responsibility of the Afghan Army. Very quickly after they found the lost Romanian,

they gave the "all unmistakable." I discovered that a 107mm rocket affected a few hundred yards away close to the helicopter arrival zone. Once more, there were no wounds or harm, and this affirmed the insight that the foe was ineffectual in terminating their rockets.

The senior authority in Gardez was booked to get back to the states soon, and the majority of them didn't have Combat Action Badges. They utilized this occasion to present countless Combat Action Badge demands, and my name was on the program. The honor models for the Combat Action Badge was: locked in by the adversary or drawing in the foe in an unfriendly country. The Combat Action Badge standards didn't characterize distances nor characterize "being locked in" by the foe; thusly, there were various understandings of rules necessities among commandants and leaders.

The usually perceived distance models were inside the shoot span of a side of the road bomb or mortar/rocket assault. The shoot span of a 107mm rocket is 12.5 yards. For this situation, the detailed rocket sway area was the helicopter arrival zone region, which would have been something like 400 yards away, making this Combat Action Badge capability occasion sketchy. At that point, I was happy to be on the list and granted the Combat Action Badge as I didn't have a clue what activity I would insight later on. Looking back, in the wake of encountering a few additional passing occasions, I feel a little embarrassed that the honor date of my Combat Action Badge was this rocket assault. I feel respected and special to wear the Combat Action Badge after this organization as I felt like I procured it a few times over and did not depend on a misrepresented attack.

Since our corps and detachment base camp were on the somewhat protected base, there was a ton of talk and show about finish of-visit grants, Combat Action Badges, and battle patches, particularly for those returning home soon. There were a wide range of tales about the Bronze Star grant, including standards, number of missions, and openness to risk. The vast majority of the troopers wanted a Bronze Star decoration as it is a battle grant, however individuals frequently misrepresented their activities to fit the rules. We heard gossipy tidbits about individuals being granted the Bronze Star despite the fact that they were terminated from their work. The conversations in regards to battle patches were more emotional, particularly without clear guidelines, and our counselor task was to a team. The overall direction was that we could wear the battle fix of Combined Forces Command – Afghanistan since Task Force Phoenix nor the Transition Command had patches. Most battle counselors didn't wear a battle fix on their arrangement in light of the fact that various pioneers would have various assessments on what was authorized.

After long stretches of leading designated spots in Terra Pass, preparing the Romanians, and yet again positioning preparation, the initial segment of our force at last left on May 21st. The gathering comprised of Gross and myself, six Romanian counselors, a few translators, and a little more than 100 Afghan Army officers. We got a punctured tire on our weapon truck on the way and Gross, and I encountered a tire change, and I figured out how huge and weighty a firearm truck tire is contrasted with a normal tire. The arrangement was to head to Bermel without anyone else. In any case, the Marine battle counsel and a portion of their Afghan Army fighters met us about an hour outside Bermel. They gained adversary radio transmissions demonstrating that the foe would set up a trap on our escort. The foe didn't wind up assaulting us as we had excessively enormous of a component with the additional help. We halted at the boundary control highlight drop off Gross, a Romanian guide, and some Afghan Army troopers, and afterward drove for two hours to show up at Bermel. It was an extremely drawn out day, and we didn't get to bed in the transient B-Hut until exceptionally late that night.

We spent the following not many days chatting with the Marine battle guides and getting orientated with the space. We went on a couple of watches with the Marine battle consultant and their Afghan Army officers through Malaksay, Marghah, and appropriated philanthropic guide in Mangratay. On May 24th, we led a mounted watch into the close by mountains, and we got off to move to the highest point of the mountain. To diminish weight moving to the highest point of the 10,000+ foot mountain, I followed the extreme Marines and eliminated my body protective layer plates and another stuff. We gradually wound our direction to the top, going over rock edges and adjusting on an exceptionally thin way. I was unable to pause and rest, and my muscles stressed. After arriving at the culmination, we found a vacant perception present as there showed up on have been battling positions with rock dividers. Looking back, we were lucky that the perception post was empty as we as a whole were generally depleted and left our protection plates and other stuff at the lower part of the mountain. The perspectives from the highest point of the mountain were staggering and definitely worth the ascension. It was practically harder to go down the mountain than going up as gravity and lose ground cover needed you to get you to the base a lot quicker than you hoped.

We visited the line control point the day after our mountain observation. Gross invested the majority of his energy in Shkin however would be at the boundary control point frequently, and the conditions at the line control point were horrifying. During our visit to the boundary control point, a couple of us needed to stroll across the line to the Pakistan designated spot. There was a discussion assuming that was a smart thought, and we chose to stroll over without the additional body protective layer to introduce less of a hostile power. We took a few photos of our illicit line crossing and immediately headed back.

ur development party Romanian counsels conversed with the other Romanian consultants in Gardez with worries about the adversary danger around Bermel. The Marine battle counsels had a full supplement of firearm trucks with weighty weapons. Interestingly, a large portion of the Romanians would be in pickups with AK-47s, and there was discussion about the Romanian country understanding that wouldn't leave them alone in this threatening region. The administration chose to trade the Afghan Army legions and keep the Marine battle counsels in Bermel and keep the Romanian guides in Gardez. With this change, there wasn't a prerequisite for as numerous US counselors with the Romanians. Since the other official consultant had marked the hand receipts, administration chose to keep him with the Romanian counselor and uproot Gross and me. These progressions caused gigantic disappointment since all of this occurred in the re-positioning, and presently, we didn't have a task. Following a couple of days and a few escorts through Gardez, Gross and I were reassigned to battle support consultants in Sharana.

ROCKETS RED GLARE

"Bombs rushing in air." – Star Spangled Banner

I spent a lot of time the first couple of weeks sitting in the operations center on staff duty, and I had a couple of patrols and convoys to start to get familiar with the surrounding area. Since I was familiar with computer organizing, I set up the organization associations for the unit tasks focus so it would be prepared when they showed up. I didn't invest a lot of energy with the past official and the mounted guns organization, however I gave receipt our firearm truck and weapons. The Afghan Army ordnance organization got two D-30 howitzers the month earlier, yet haven't directed any cannons preparing as they have been leading watches and designated spots. The D-30 howitzer is a 122mm towed howitzer that requires a group of eight warriors to fire five 45-pound adjusts each moment up to 9.6 miles. Gross was expecting to be the surveillance organization battle counselor. He didn't establish a decent connection with the contingent group pioneer as he failed to remember his rifle in Gardez during our caravans. Gross in the long run moved to one more infantry regiment after two or three weeks.

My firearm truck was viewed as the best weapon truck as it had a substantial automatic rifle, a strategic satellite radio, a high-recurrence radio, electronic counter-measures, and a speaker for an iPod. We had a grouping of star bunches, thermite explosives, claymore mine, AT-4 enemy of tank weapon (84mm unguided, versatile, single-shot recoilless weapon), additional protection penetrating ammo and an expendable AK-47. I don't remember where the AK-47 came from or how we got it, yet it was planned to be accessible for our translator or battle consultants in case we got into an enormous fight. We never removed our AK-47 from its stockpiling spot in the firearm truck.

On June seventh, there was a dire message to stock and give an account of against tank weapons as one of the detachment consultant groups detailed one missing. The letter demonstrated an examination was beginning, and the sergeant dependable may have monetary responsibility for the weapon. All things considered, there was likewise a high worry that the adversary may find it and use it against us. It was not unexpected practice to utilize the tie of the counter tank weapon to connect to the open bring forth in the heavy armament specialist's station of the firearm truck, and they presumed that this enemy of tank weapon wasn't safely joined and tumbled off of the firearm truck during a caravan. On June fourteenth, I helped a unit counselor to change over the examination report into .pdf design. I saw that a nearby public tracked down the counter tank weapon and gave it to a strategic human insight specialist on June twelfth, who returned it to the unit group pioneer. The exploring official suggested a letter of censure against the sergeant who lost responsibility of the counter tank weapon. I would ultimately wind up going on certain missions with this sergeant.

It was the evening of June sixteenth, and it was getting blistering in eastern Afghanistan, however our room had a Chico forced air system, which kept the temperature fair inside. I was dozing on a brief bunk worked of 2x4s in my shorts and a shirt within sheets and a light cover. I was simply alloted to this unit for under about fourteen days and anticipated moving bunks the following day. A huge touchy sound woke me up at roughly 1:00 am, immediately trailed by another. It was dull in the room without windows, and I heard somebody outside shouting "approaching." My prompt idea was to get to the dugout as fast as could be expected. I put on my glasses, boots without my socks, body defensive layer, head protector, and gun. While I was snatching my stuff, I heard my bunkmates preparing as well, and I had musings of beating them to the dugout, similar to an unannounced race. Before I planned to leave, I understood that it was in the evening, so I better snatch my night vision goggles, which I immediately looked for in my backpack and put them on, which would be my first time since sending preparing. I was quick to leave our room, and I hustled down the 20-yard long rear entryway to the bunker.

Once I got inside the shelter, I believed that I had a fast reaction as there were just two obscure translators inside. I had dominated my fanciful race. As I crouched inside for a couple of seconds, I saw no other individual was coming into the dugout, and my psyche started dashing to attempt to think where every other person would have gone. I chose to pass on the haven to find my mounted guns sergeant counsel. I left the shelter, and I returned down the resting quarter's back street. Traveling through the back street, I didn't see anybody, and I began seeing the hints of fight with more programmed gunfire, blasts, and blasts. I really look at our room, and there was no one inside. I started to freeze, earnestly needing to find another person, and I believed I was abandoned and all alone.

I felt that possibly the counselors previously headed toward the Afghan Army side to assist with planning the protection, so I raced through the little open door. I went a short far beyond the entry and saw some Afghan Army officers going around and going into a steel trailer to get more ammunition with my night vision. I entered the confusion of mass conflict and had more frenzy as I didn't see anybody I perceived. More tracers hummed overhead with stronger blasts. I felt like an outsider in a weird land. I could see with the night vision goggles, yet the Afghan Army couldn't see me. We were unable to impart. I had no clue about what to do, however I realized that I would have rather not be on this side of the Afghan Army base.

For each tracer round, there are four customary projectiles that you can't see. Tracers are projectiles that consume a substance on the cartridge that enlightens during its flight. Tracer adjusts are regularly stacked as each fifth round, and help the shooter's point, particularly during evening time. In any case, a tracer round will likewise recognize the shooter's situation to the enemy.

I ran back to the US compound, however I didn't go through the rear entryway once more. I went towards our little leaving region where we had our about six firearm trucks left. I saw one of the vehicles running, and a US fighter was stacking the automatic rifle on the top. I was eased to some degree that I tracked down somebody. I understood that they were taking the weapon truck out so the huge entryway would need to get opened, so I ran back to the entry. I felt hurried to open the latch as the weapon truck was coming, and I needed to have the door open. I battled to see the numbers on the latch with my night vision goggles, and I was amazingly disappointed with myself since I didn't have my electric lamp to have the option to see the lock. I was wearing my actual wellness uniform, and I normally kept my spotlight in my fight uniform coat pocket. I surged up to the driver and said that I was unable to get the entryway open and required a spotlight. Individual Wisconsin official counselor Larson had an electric lamp and assisted me with opening the lock and open the metal door. Just after the weapon truck passed through the entryway, an enormous touchy sound was exceptionally close, and Larson said something with the impact of "Blessed crap."

I needed to extend the picture of a more battle experienced official, so I immediately let him know that it should be the Afghan Army discharging their cannons. Larson said we ought to return to the activities place for cover and discover what is happening. I immediately concurred however felt enormous inward embarrassment as I never contemplated going to the activities community. As we began towards the activities place, I asked why I let Larson know that the touchy sound was Afghan Army ordnance. As the gunnery battle counselor, I realized that the Afghan Army didn't have the ammo to discharge their howitzers.

Once Larson and I went into the activities place, it was extremely splendid with the lights on, and there were twelve individuals inside a tumultuous room with individuals talking, hollering, and on the radios. I remained close to the entryway, and no one asked where I was for sure I was doing. I was the just one in shorts and shirt as others were in varieties of our fight garbs. One of the pioneers requested volunteers to bring more firearm trucks to position around the external border. I was coordinated to a firearm truck with two detachment consultants to be the driver, which was great since I didn't have my uniform, rifle and other stuff. The three of us went to the weapon truck, and I headed to a spot on the eastern border. I was unable to see over the HESCO divider, yet the heavy armament specialist said he had the option to. At this point in the assault, the gunfire and blasts diminished. We sat in our weapon truck, attempting to sort out what was happening by the radio reports.

e got called to return and informed we could tolerate downing. I left the firearm truck, and we returned to the activities place with the automatic weapon. We could return to our quarters, and we would have an after-activity report meeting at some point during the day. I returned to my bunk, needing to rest since I was anticipating visiting on the web with my significant other toward the beginning of the day. Toward the start of the organization, I decided not to educate my better half regarding the terrible things to decrease her concern, so I needed to be certain that I was conscious for our visit session.

We had a short group meeting the next day about by and large what occurred, however wound up being a conversation to build up a battle guide night watch, or base security power. The day after the assault, we had a guard mission to drop off certain guides and get some new ones. I saw an email half a month after the fact that showed that the assault went on for around 40 minutes and that there were roughly 30 mortars. Rocket-moved projectiles and automatic rifle discharge came from various areas, and that there was some underlying harm to a portion of the compressed wood building and our treadmill. The messages portrayed how a gathering of consultants went to the highest point of the restrooms

to set up perception. A gathering of battle consultants set up the activities community and called higher central command on the radios. One more gathering of counselors reacted in the weapon trucks. During this assault, my first real commitment, I understood I was ill-equipped. I expected to establish a decent connection with my new group. Starting the following day, I ensured that my uniform and hardware were spread out in a specific order.

Beyond the brief time frame of feeling amazingly disengaged during this assault, there was not some other time where I was separated from everyone else for the whole organization. There was consistently somebody around, giving definitely no protection. It was difficult to settle on telephone decisions home on the grounds that there were others inside two feet. We utilized light covers to make dividers around our bunks, yet they don't impede commotion and just to some degree encompassed the bed.

The remainder of June and the main seven day stretch of July were really lethargic. I finished an infrequent mission and a couple escorts. Amusingly, we were on an escort to Gardez to put in new electronic counter-measures on our firearm trucks, and we had a side of the road bomb assault coming. The adversary covered a high touchy mortar shell in a soil hill in some street development. The side of the road bomb exploded behind our last firearm truck in our little escort and didn't bring on any harm or wounds Advantageously, we had an Afghan Army watch with their battle guide exceptionally nearby, and they confined a speculated hitman.

It appeared as though I was on the base security power list more than any other individual. Since our base assault, not set in stone that we really wanted a battle guide presence at the front door during the evening. We would drive a weapon truck onto a little slope close to the primary entry, and utilize our thermals and night vision goggles to give further perception. We could guarantee that the Afghan Army troopers worked the entryway appropriately. There weren't set up occasions for base security power to stay away from consistency, yet for the most part began among supper and nightfall and finished between 2:00 am and dawn. Base security power obligation messed up rest plans. In case you were on a base security drive, you should have the morning off to rest, yet as a general rule, there were gatherings or mission necessities that forestalled the rest. Being on the base security power was exceptionally dull, and I was happy we had the iPod speaker in our weapon truck. I couldn't say whether the base security power was a contributing variable, however the foe didn't assault our base again.

On July seventh, we held a short commemoration administration for a previous battle counsel, SGM Jeffery McLochlin of Indiana National Guard, who was killed by little arms discharge close to Orgun-E on July fifth. SGM McLochlin was

recently allocated as a battle support counselor and afterward reassigned to an Afghan Army infantry contingent. I had not known SGM McLochlin, yet a couple of others in Sharana had known him. SGM McLochlin was an Army Ranger with more than 19 years of military help and was a cop in Plymouth, IN.

The day after our dedication administration, I had a short meeting with Meg Jones, a correspondent from the Milwaukee Journal Sentinel paper, on a speedy nation visit for stories from Wisconsin warriors. The story, Guts, indeed, however warriors likewise need an arrangement, was distributed on July eighth, 2006, and she cited me with respect to the measure of Afghan Army fighters leave and their terminating precision. Meg Jones composed five reports on our Wisconsin consultant team.

On July ninth, I was amped up for going on leave soon, so I went through the day pressing. We had a short mission from 9:00 – 11:00 pm to look through some mud-walled Afghan homes toward the south of our base as there was an insight report demonstrating that there might be a weapons store. It was one more mediocre mission as I helped the Afghan Army unit pioneer with security on the edge and got back to base.

Around 12 PM, we were made aware of react as a speedy response power to an adversary assault on an Afghan Police station at the boundary of Ghazni and Paktika areas. Our central goal had six battle counsels in two weapon trucks and around 24 Afghan Army and their pickups. The arrangement was to leave promptly since the assault was progressing, connect up with an Afghan Police component in Sharana and race to the guide of the Afghan Police station. I was driving, Ressler was working the substantial assault rifle, sergeant counselor Steward was in the front seat, and our mediator, Obie, was in the back front seat. Ressler set up the automatic rifle, and I was directing radio checks while Steward was preparing the Afghan Army fighters. Our weapon truck just got another electronic counter-measures framework, and it was fundamental to get the radio checks finished prior to initiating the electronic counter-measures as it would meddle with our radio transmissions also. We got the order to go, go, go. Along these lines, we went. I initiated the electronic counter-measures, and we left our base. Two Afghan Police pickups were looking out for the primary street in Sharana to assist with directing us to the Afghan Police station.

One of the framework projects was clearing streets inside the nation, and they nearly finished the course from Sharana to Ghazni. We cruised all over the blockades and had the option to drive sensibly quick down the recently cleared street. Not very far past the hindrances, we ran over an Afghan cop who had lost his weapon and fled from the Afghan Police station to get away. He got into the rear of one of the Afghan Police pickups. While halted, Ressler saw he was unable to see the other firearm truck. We attempted to connect with our other weapon truck or base, yet our electronic counter-measures probably meddled with the sign. We chose to keep the electronic counter-gauges on and proceed with our main goal. I was driving with my night vision goggles, following the Afghan Police pickup, and began struggling seeing because of a brilliant light ahead.

There wasn't sufficient noticeable light to see without night vision goggles, yet the light was adequately splendid to clean out the night vision. Steward chose to descent and direct a straight methodology with the Afghan Army officers and Afghan Police. While Steward was endeavoring to get everybody in position, Ressler found that we didn't have the necessary headspace and timing system to emplace the weighty automatic weapon into functional mode, and would simply have the option to discharge each round in turn. We began moving gradually forward, and afterward, the Afghan Army fighters beginning terminating their AK-47s and dispatched several rocket-impelled explosives. The rocket-pushed projectiles headed to the overall bearing of the light. In any case, the AK-47 tracers went towards the light to practically straight in the sky. I don't accept the "Inshalla" terminating strategy is viable. After a serious, short volley, the terminating halted. It appeared to be that all the shooting was towards the light, and we didn't get any shooting consequently. We gradually proceeded with the development toward the light. At the point when we showed up at the light and Afghan Police station, the adversary was no more. The structure was slug ridden, and an Afghan Police pickup was projectile ridden and was ablaze. We were in the blink of an eye joined by the other firearm truck when we showed up at the Afghan Police station. The battle counselors in the other weapon truck thought the most dire outcome imaginable as they couldn't contact us on the radio and saw the shoot and tracers. We utilized our weapon truck for overwatch, and the Afghan Army led a breadth around the space. We held one more watch to the Afghan Police station the following day for an appraisal of fight damage.

NON-STANDARD MISSIONS

"It's not the size of the canine in the battle, it's the size of the battle in the canine." – Mark Twain

It took 42 days for me to take my two-week leave period. Backward planning was necessary to make sure you are at Bagram before your flight departs, and there are often delays with convoys and flights. I had a escort to Zormat on July sixteenth, changed to one more guard to Gardez where I put in several days, changed to one more caravan to Camp Phoenix, and afterward a ride with workers for hire toward the rear of a shielded Suburban to Bagram on July twentieth. The departure from Bagram on July 22nd was on a fly freight plane with front seats introduced and was a wonderful flight, however I felt my stomach drop as the stream freight plane rehearsed a battle arrival with exceptionally unexpected drops and tough maneuvers upon appearance in Kuwait. After handling, the pilot said that the external temperature was 124 degrees Fahrenheit at 4:30 pm, and it seemed like a hot pass dryer strolling over the incline. The following day, we left Kuwait in a contracted non military personnel rotator trip to Atlanta, GA, with a two-hour delay in Germany. I was on a standard outing from Atlanta to Milwaukee on July 24th. I voyaged as far as possible home in my uniform and got a great deal of acknowledgment at the air terminals; nonetheless, with voyaging and transient, I was worn out, and I didn't feel sufficiently clean to be marched around. My significant other got me the air terminal in Milwaukee. It was dreamlike to be home in Wisconsin, and it was so magnificent to see green grass and trees, and voyaging quicker than 20 miles each hour on genuine roads.

My significant other and I had two or three unique occasions arranged and had some customary exercises, for example, going to the Department of Motor Vehicles, trimming the grass and cleaning the house. We went to Wisconsin Dells twice to go on the stream boats and scaled down golf and once for the day at Mt Olympus Waterpark. We went to my old neighborhood to go on a barge boat ride with my family while heading to Door County. We remained at a retreat in Door County and delighted in supper in our room and going plane skiing. I have never been on a Jet Ski, and we had it for two hours. We alternated driving and circumvented Sturgeon Bay and saw a portion of the "tall boats." It was just no time like the present to return the Jet Ski, and I was driving. Shockingly, as I pivoted to go to the dock, I controlled too sharp, going excessively lethargic, and spilled. I had a hell of time endeavoring to turn the Jet Ski over, and we discovered that the dry compartment doesn't remain dry when submerged. I had my advanced camera in the compartment yet had the option to get it dried to work once more. We went through a day at the Wisconsin State Fair and went to the firecrackers at Riverfest in Watertown. I needed to partake in the firecrackers yet couldn't delay until they got done, possibly on the grounds that I had quite recently experienced genuine blasts a littlc while prior.

It was early morning on August ninth at 6:20 am for my return departure from Milwaukee to Atlanta. Bidding farewell to my better half the subsequent time was a lot harder, and I would have rather not return. Military faculty getting back from leave met at the USO office in the air terminal in Atlanta. When they represented everybody, they marched us through the air terminal, with the groups applauding and cheering. We had a contracted business departure from Atlanta, through Germany, back to Kuwait. I went through two days in Kuwait because of flight abrogations lastly traveled to Bagram on August twelfth. I should be on a Chinook helicopter flight the following day, yet they knock me, and I went through a little more than seven days in Bagram in transient status. Other than investing a great deal of energy strolling around, I watched numerous motion pictures in the USO. A few Soldiers appreciated transient time by resting or perusing. I felt like I expected to accomplish something, however there wasn't a thing to do, and it was a battle to remain somewhat involved. I was at last ready to show for a Chinook helicopter ride at 2:30 am on August 21st. A Chinook helicopter CH-47 Boeing airplane is a twin-motor, couple rotor, substantial lift helicopter intended to convey 40 prepared fighters or 24,000 pounds of freight. This helicopter has a scope of 460 miles at 180 miles each hour, and generally has medium assault rifles mounted as an afterthought entryway.

This airplane has unrivaled execution in the high mountain elevations. A unit counsel group got me from the Sharana

Provincial Reconstruction Team to return to Sharana.

Upon return, Ressler and I began big guns preparing, yet Ressler had his leave booked, and I was entrusted to offer help on another mission. The Afghan Army troopers at Orgun-E were arranging a huge scope clear mission in the Pir Kowti valley with support from Task Force Catamount and unit Afghan Army central command. We left for Orgun-E on August 29th for two evenings for an arranging meeting. At the point when we showed up, we got the mission brief. The following day when the base camp staff proceeded with their preparation, I went with an Afghan Army infantry unit consultant group to lead traffic light focuses the entire day in the downpour. We had course freedom support that found and annihilated eight separate side of the road bombs, making our drive back to Orgun-E extremely extensive. We directed an escort back to Sharana the following day.

While we were gone, Sharana got a portable kitchen trailer and two US Navy food administration staff to get ready breakfast and supper dinners. After a little difficulty setting up the trailer, the Navy prepares warmed semi-arranged suppers on the burner units and served the dinners on the trailer, so we didn't have to alternate cooking on the fire any longer. I couldn't partake in this foodservice much as I was in Sharana for a negligible time frame among missions and my next assignment.

I remained in Sharana for two evenings before we led an escort back to Orgun-E to execute the Pir Kowti mission. While at Orgun-E, I got a short class from the Task Force Catamount mortar segment on the 120mm mortar, and I was expecting to have the option to shoot a mortar round. Steward and I were the battle counsels for around 15 Afghan Army troopers, and our piece of the mission was to give a security component to the Task Force Catamount 120mm mortar area. The arrangement was to air attack the security component and the mortar segment onto a mountain ridge outside of the scope region to give fire backing and concentrate by Chinook helicopters in several days.

The Afghan Army officers directed practices for section and exit on the back incline of a Chinook helicopter during the evening. We stacked the Chinook helicopters and took off from Orgun-E into the evening. The addition point was a few miles away, yet the Chinook helicopters zoomed around for some time to give trickery. Shockingly, when we handled, my legs nodded off as I hunched on my backpack close to the incline of the Chinook helicopter, which made my exit troublesome. While I was holding up for my legs to awaken, I saw that we weren't the first to arrive.

he Afghan Army warrior security component should be embedded first and afterward the mortar area on the second Chinook helicopter. We landed second as the mortar area was at that point there. With this disarray, working with night vision, and simply getting orientated, I experienced issues getting coordinated. Steward started to lead the pack in emplacing the Afghan Army troopers to guarantee edge security. Steward and I set up a situation on the edge security that would permit phenomenal perceivability of Pir Kowti valley. I remained alert to allow Steward to get some rest. We go through the following two days doing spot keeps an eye on the Afghan Army officers to guarantee they remained alert. There was very little confidence that the Afghan Army troopers would give reasonable security, so Steward and I felt like we expected to enhance insurance. This mission immediately transformed into an exhausting experience. The mortar segment terminated one light round on the principal morning to set the mortar base plate, and an Afghan Army officer told me the best way to choose seeds from an obscure plant. Feeling the feeling of obligation, I didn't rest during the day and didn't rest soundly the subsequent evening and wound up with five hours of rest more than 60 hours. We rcmovcd at dinnertime on the subsequent day, and I immediately went to bed.

n September eighth, we led a caravan to get back to Sharana with 13 Afghan Army pickups and three weapon trucks, and I was in the guard. I was the medium heavy weapons specialist, Steward was the driver, and we had two unit counsels as travelers. We left Orgun-E early in the day, and it was hot, radiant, and dry. We were depleted, yet had an uplifting outlook as our air attack mission was successful.

Usually, when my sergeant and I went on missions, we would put the radios on the speakers and didn't utilize the radio framework. On this caravan mission, Steward needed to utilize the radio framework, so we both wore headsets. Notwithstanding the radio headsets, I put on earbuds with iPod music on a low volume to keep me engaged and conscious. Close to partially through our two-hour drive back to Sharana, our reality was shaken as I paid attention to Alanis Morrissette. We were on a dusty country road going through some tough slopes, simply adjusting a slight bend. Kaboom!

The following activity I review is cresting over the highest point of the back bring forth and seeing just dark and dark smoke, and Steward inquiring as to whether I am alright. I answered that I was unable to see anyone behind me. Steward halted the firearm truck, pivoted, and went to the blast site. I was confounded with regards to what simply occurred and what I ought to do. I was worried about turning around

in light of the fact that there may be more side of the road bombs. Someone said something regarding a hitman on the radio, and Steward hollered about charging the assault rifle. I stacked the medium automatic rifle however had no idea where to search for the enemy.

Steward halted the weapon truck barely shy of the blast site, near where we were the point at which the blast occurred. There was as yet dim smoke gradually floating away, with an extraordinary and indefinable smell: the smell consolidated blast buildup, consuming elastic, tissue, and residue. The hood of the pickup was behind us, showing that it probably blew past us in the blast. There was a ravaged, ridiculous body lying in the country road close to a little cavity. I didn't see it promptly, yet the pickup was topsy turvy, contiguous and easy from now on street, behind an enormous stone formation.

ther battle consultants, Afghan Army officers, and Steward immediately went to the obliterated pickup with their battle lifeline packs to deliver medical aid. Steward acknowledged we wanted a more significant security region, so he requested that an official counselor help the Afghan Army to push out the security edge. In the mean time, I kept on working my assault rifle, assisting with security. I remained in the firearm truck without help from anyone else in wonder concerning how much annihilation happened. I was inside the impact and bits of the pickup shot past me. I was attempting to justify why I was not harmed or even killed. Maybe on the grounds that I am more limited, so less of me is uncovered, or I am super-quick and can avoid the way.

The counselors did their clinical not really set in stone to require a medevac Blackhawk helicopter to endeavor to save a couple of the lives. Steward returned hurrying to the firearm truck and had a go at calling Orgun-E. He was fruitless because of distance and slopes, and he immediately considered utilizing a convenient satellite radio recieving wire. He had the option to interface, and he mentioned a medevac and gave a circumstance report. He gave me the radio handset so he could set up the arrival zone. I kept on working the automatic weapon, hanging tight for the Blackhawk helicopter. The Afghan Army warriors and battle counsels fired tidying up the space, starting to recuperate the annihilated vehicle and help them. I addressed the radio call from the medevac, affirming our area and shade of the smoke signal. After the medevac left, it appeared to consume a huge chunk of time to get things tidied up. The Afghan Army was utilizing different pickups to drag the obliterated vehicle nearer to the street. I don't know who brought it up, but rather there was a worry for auxiliary side of the road bombs, despite the fact that individuals have been strolling around the space. Somebody called for

Explosive Ordinance Disposal (EOD) support from Sharana Provincial Reconstruction Team, yet it would require them a few hours to get to our area. The Afghan Army required a wrecker truck to get the harmed pickup. Egotistically, I was becoming baffled with regards to what amount of time this is requiring, as I without a doubt needed to return to my bed and continue on from this occasion.

Ultimately, the dangerous law removal group showed up. One officer put on the dangerous security suit and checked the pit region. He informed us there were two other dangerous gadgets covered in the street. The dangerous specialists cleared the region, set a charge, and blew different gadgets set up. A huge jingle truck showed up and winched the harmed pickup into its truck bed. Night-time at the site, we were prepared to continue our guard. Our weapon truck needed to leave the guard and stop at Sharana Provincial Reconstruction Team to have a project worker download our information in light of the fact that our firearm truck had the electronic counter-measures close to thc blast. After he ran his program, he let Steward and I in on that the side of the road bomb was remotely set off and that our electronic counter-measures postponed the start until it passed our "defensive air pocket." It was great to realize that the electronic counter-measures deferred the explosion of the side of the road bomb to ensure us. Shockingly, the electronic counter-gauges just postponed the blast and didn't secure the vehicle behind us. I might have had a limited drink that evening in festival of life and to quiet down. As a topography illustration, Pálinka is a customary organic product cognac from the Romania space of the world. One of the Afghan Army killed was the Brigade Command Sergeant Major, the top enrolled sergeant for the Afghan Army unit commander.

fter my sending, I discovered that Steward was an unmistakable blogger and composed an extensive article about this side of the road bomb assault. The one thing that struck me in his blog was his explanation that he inquired as to whether I was OK, and I just recollect once. I possibly had a gentle blackout, and the shoot constrained me into the incubate. I had a cerebral pain that evening, yet I thought it was because of the absence of rest and drying out. Since I wasn't actually harmed, there was not a remotely good excuse to medevac me for clinical consideration. Our little battle consultant groups didn't have clinical staff. Did I have a gentle blackout? I don't know as this was before gentle awful mind injury awareness.

Within 48 hours of the side of the road bomb assault, I was once again at it once more. We spent the brief time frame cleaning weapons and vehicles, dozing, and having some close to home vacation. Our brigade group pioneer gave us a mission brief

the after a long time after our rest day. There was insight that a presumed self destruction aircraft expected to kill the neighborhood Afghan area lead representative. There was a specific worry to stay away from one more assault on our base as the lead representative's complicated was nearby our central command. The regiment group pioneer split us into four gatherings to direct a "check-watch shrub" mission with some Afghan Army officers. I was a mounted guns official, and I was certifiably not an educated authority on infantry strategies, yet I never known about a "check-watch shrubbery" mission. Sergeant counselor Glidden and I would be the principle component with Obie and weapon truck with the medium assault rifle, and 15 Afghan Army fighters in three pickups. Steward and the unit tasks official counselor would be with

30 Afghan Army warriors for the speedy response power. Individual unit work force official counselor Weist and his colleague would leave the base and set up an overwatch position on Bataana Hill, a little slope several hundred yards northwest of our base that the Afghan Army utilized for a perception post. Weist would have a weapon truck with the weighty assault rifle and warm sight. In principle, there was potential to see traffic from two or three miles from this vantage point. Our regiment group pioneer remained in his quarters on the base to screen the radios.

A "check-watch bramble" would be a mix of a presence watch, a designated spot, and a trap. The idea is withdraw the base at dull in vehicles with our lights on for a presence watch. When we traveled with regards to a mile in the dry waterway bed, we would wind down the lights, go calm, and build up a snare position. To decide whether somebody passing through the dry stream bed was companion or enemy, an unexpected designated spot group would leap out of their concealing spots. On the off chance that they were the adversary or the presumed self destruction aircraft, we would have the trap team.

Glidden was the sergeant battle counsel to the central command organization. I was the official battle counsel to the big guns organization. We haven't cooperated beforehand; additionally, neither Glidden nor I have worked with the Afghan Army observation leader, and we didn't have the foggiest idea about his fighters. We directed the mission brief with the observation leader and led pre-battle checks with the officers after the supper feast. At roughly 7:30 pm, we left the base with one weapon truck and three pickups with our lights on to the dry stream bed and drove south in the dry waterway bed for about a mile to a site where we could build up the trap designated spot site. Glidden encouraged the surveillance authority to set up perception focuses on the far north and south sides of our situation, to set up a solid overwatch

position which could be utilized for the trap, assign a designated spot group, and to guarantee security. While the Afghan Army surveillance leader was situating his officers, Glidden and I posted the weapon truck in an overwatch position close to the Afghan Army overwatch. Around 30 minutes subsequent to showing up on location, we gave our lattice area to the unit group pioneer and Weist in Bataana Hill.

The legion group pioneer inquired as to whether he could distinguish us, and he answered that he proved unable. The regiment group pioneer trained Glidden to streak our headlights so Weist could recognize us from Bataana Hill. I radioed the brigade group pioneer and Weist that we were around two miles to the immediate south of Bataana Hill and gave our matrix arranges once more. The contingent group pioneer actually demanded that we streak our headlights...three times for Weist to recognize us outwardly. Possible, the contingent group pioneer needed to guarantee that Weist knew where we were so he wouldn't draw in us with the substantial assault rifle; notwithstanding, after showing up at the snare site, we wound down all lights and went into a calm mode to set up for the trap. With delay, we consented and streaked our headlights multiple times, however Weist actually couldn't distinguish us. I could just see the highest point of the radio pinnacle on Bataana Hill and couldn't see the base; along these lines, it would be fairly improbable that Weist would have the option to see us. The regiment group pioneer guided us to streak our headlights multiple times once more. Once more, Weist couldn't distinguish us. The brigade group pioneer taught us to move the vehicle to higher ground and glimmer the lights three additional occasions. All things considered, with dithering, we moved our firearm truck around 15 yards to a somewhat higher spot. After we moved, we streaked our lights once more, and Weist at last expressed he could see faint flashes.

Things were getting calm, and we were sitting tight for traffic in the dry riverbed. After a brief time, the contingent group pioneer began radio informing the current football scores like clockwork. He had a TV in his room and thought it was a confidence sponsor. Glidden and I expressed we couldn't have cared less with regards to the scores since we were on a mission. The unit group pioneer kept refreshing scores on the radio, and I at last turned the radio volume down. At roughly 11:00 pm, the Sharana Provincial Reconstruction Team began directing mortar light missions. The mortar rounds' brightening was adequately close to see our vehicles and faculty around our trap site apparently. We reached our brigade group pioneer that the Provincial Reconstruction Team was enlightening our position. We were observing the Provincial Reconstruction Team radio net and heard

the message from the Provincial Reconstruction Team's battle counsel base camp, expressing that they were enlightening our region. The Provincial Reconstruction Team answered that the enlightenments were six miles toward the south of us; subsequently, they couldn't be enlightening our position. I got in the Provincial Reconstruction Team radio net and expressed that the enlightenments were not exactly a large portion of a mile toward the south of our space and gave my lattice area. The Provincial Reconstruction Team dropped their light missions.

Approximately 30 minutes after the enlightenment disaster, there were numerous shots to our nearby right, trailed by the Afghan Army rapidly bringing fire back. Glidden quickly radioed the circumstance report to our brigade group pioneer, who educated us to remain in our position and not to move. We were in defilade in the riverbed, and there was not an unmistakable shot to the foe powers, so I discharged a few suppressive adjusts overhead with the medium assault rifle. The gunfire immediately eased back and halted. Glidden not set in stone that we want to escape the defilade to the strategic position 20 yards to one side. We moved the weapon truck into the new position. When we moved into place, the terminating proceeded once more, however at a somewhat further distance. We calculated that a few foes came around the bend of the mud-walled Afghan home to one side and saw the Afghan Army pickup and our weapon truck and began drawing in with their AK-47s. The Afghan Army started to seek after the foe however immediately withdrew after the foe moved several hundred yards away. The legion group pioneer alarmed Steward and the speedy response power to react to our guide. Be that as it may, in evident Afghan Army design, the greater part of the Afghan Army officers weren't prepared nor close by the pickups. There was an extended deferral getting the Afghan Army fast response power moving, and they left the base with something like 15 officers rather than the 30 soldiers.

meanwhile, at the snare site, it hushed up once more. We were experiencing issues getting a status from the Afghan Army surveillance leader and guaranteeing that he kept up with security. Glidden, Obie, and I were getting extremely disappointed, endeavoring to deal with the Afghan Army officers, building up responsibility, and guaranteeing that we kept up with security. The fast response power showed up, and we radioed Steward a refreshed circumstance report. The quick response power began toward the foe withdrawal, not really set in stone that the adversary got away by means of cruisers and were as of now not nearby. Glidden was frantically working with the Afghan Army observation leader to acquire security, however the Afghan Army surveillance commandant was resistant.

nce the speedy response power got back to our position, they took positions on the back area to set up security. We speculated the close by mud-walled Afghan home for helping the adversary assault on our area. The force group pioneer needed it looked by the Afghan Police and have our Afghan Army leading security around the mud-walled Afghan home. We as a whole remained in our edge security for right around two hours before the Afghan Police at long last showed up to look through the mud-walled Afghan home, which brought about nothing. The all-unmistakable was given, and we got back to the base at around 4:30 am without any wounds or harm to any US or Afghan Army work force or hardware. We later discovered that the foe that evening was reasonable associated with the area lead representative's besieging plan, and our activities that evening deflected an attack.

My schedule and notes alluded to this mission being led on September tenth, when the mission began. It was numerous years some other time when I understood that the firefight segment happened on September eleventh. There is a considerable amount of nostalgic worth in realizing that I discharged the medium automatic rifle in a firefight with foe powers on the morning of the fifth commemoration of the September eleventh assaults. Military vernacular for a firefight is TIC, which is the shortening for troops-in-contact.

eeping track of time was befuddling. More often than not utilized was 24-hour nearby time, however a few reports and timetables were utilizing "Zulu," Greenwich Mean Time. Afghanistan is three hours and 30 minutes in front of Zulu time and is one of a handful of the spaces on the planet to be counterbalanced by 30 mins, and they don't utilize light investment funds time. Wisconsin time would be nine and a half hours behind Afghanistan time and would change because of sunshine investment funds in Wisconsin. I had a Casio watch with hands and an advanced presentation. I utilized the hands for nearby time, the advanced presentation for Zulu time, and the resulting computerized time for Wisconsin time. These time region contrasts would make calling home more confounded with work and rest plans. I really wanted a morning timer, so I purchased a vibrating watch that I would wear around evening time. It was promoted for senior residents to help to remember drug times yet was exceptionally valuable, awakening me and keeping up with the admiration of bunkmates that would have diverse schedules.

Local wild canines around Sharana was a positive irritation and presented wellbeing concerns. Canines are not esteemed as a pet in Afghanistan and are frequently left to battle for themselves. Experiencing childhood in humble community Wisconsin, my family explored different avenues regarding a few unique pets and never had a solid association with them. We had loner crabs, fish, felines, and a canine. We got our canine from a neighborhood rancher from his litter, and he remained outside in a canine house. He developed to turn into a boisterous, yapping canine that was not entirely congenial or cherishing, and the wild canines around Sharana would help me to remember him. To kill the wild canines, a few counsels would utilize the canines s target practice from the HESCO wall.

The overall request in Afghanistan restricted canines and pets on the bases; notwithstanding, the greater part of the bases had two or three canines to associate with rat destruction and as a base mascot or pet. My flat mate in Sharana self-took on a little wild canine, and he had it rest in our room. I was certainly against this since I didn't have a clue about his medical issue, and he was not prepared so he would bite on everything. I voiced my interests a few times, yet my grumblings to our group chief disappeared rapidly. That rangy canine made pressure with a couple other advisors.

I was doled out to another mission two days following our firefight. Weist, Glidden, and I were the battle consultants with Obie for a multi-day mission. There were around 30 Afghan Army warriors in six pickups, and we were completely coordinated into Task Force Catamount components with course freedom engineer support. We as a whole arranged toward the start of the night on September thirteenth. We drove under front of obscurity for around three hours, where we set up an entry point outside the town of Miri, Andar region in the Ghazni area. I had considerations of why we were directing activities in another person's space of liability, for what reason was I connected up with these battle consultants, and why we were with these Afghan Army warriors. Since I had base security power the earlier evening and drove the greater part of this evening, I was really worn out and wound up sleeping steering the ship while we sat tight for dawn in our entry point. Glidden was the heavy weapons specialist and said he didn't nod off, thank heavens. I was as yet exhausted at sunrise, so Glidden offered me a spot of Red Man biting tobacco saying that it should assist with awakening me. It made me more ready, yet it made me exceptionally sick. Example learned –

Red Man disagrees with me.

The following three days were basically the same. The greater part of Task Force Catamount began building up a transitory base at the locale community in Miri due to having a fantastic opening and meeting of Afghan older folks in a couple of days. A portion of the Task Force Catamount components directed watches to towns around the

region to lead appraisals. These evaluations for the most part comprised of Task Force Catamount staff and the Afghan Army/battle counsel giving security. Ordinarily, we would head to the edges of a town and descent. We left some staff with the vehicles, and the rest would foot watch into the town and look for the older folks. The Task Force Catamount initiative conversed with the elderly folks about undesirable guests, what their town required, and the Afghan Army troopers gave security, and they interfaced with different individuals from the village.

fter a few hours, we would foot watch back to the vehicles and drive to the following town. Upon haziness, we set up our vehicles in a circle with the weapons bringing up and alternated resting in the soil, on top of the firearm truck, and in the firearm truck seats. I found that you could eliminate the seat-back of the firearm truck's back seats and use them to cover the footwells to make a semi-level region to rest inside the weapon truck. I rested in a camping cot and removed my boots, jeans, and coat. We utilized child wipes to tidy up toward the beginning of the day, and I utilized a battery-fueled razor to eliminate a portion of the stubble all over. Following a day in the hotness and residue, we were all damp with sweat and stinky. We had instances of water, Gatorade, MREs, a case of Pop-Tarts, and additional ammo in our trunk, with our backpacks secured on the highest point of the truck slope. Glidden generally worked the assault rifle, Weist was the essential consultant to the Afghan Army, and I was the driver and composed with the authority in Task Force Catamount.

The main occurrence during these days was on the principal day when a Task Force Catamount firearm truck struck a strain plate side of the road bomb that annihilated piece of the vehicle with practically no extreme wounds. Their weapon truck was several vehicles before us. There was radio correspondence about a presumed adversary close by, so the Afghan Army and our weapon truck set up a designated spot down a back street. Following a few hours at the designated spot, Task Force Catamount had the option to recuperate the harmed firearm truck, and we proceeded with our watches and evaluations. These days were long, hot, dry, and extraordinarily baffling. The dissatisfaction and stress weren't from the conditions... it was from the Afghan Army officers. The Afghan Army warriors would consistently not pay attention to our direction, rest during their watch, and complain.

Task Force Catamount and battle guides had night vision goggles and drove with dark out lights. The Afghan Army warriors didn't have night vision goggles, yet we educated them to painstakingly follow the "feline eyes" of

the vehicle before them. The Afghan Army drivers would frequently streak their headlights to see where they were going, disturbing everybody's vision. We furnished the Afghan Army warriors with instances of Halal dinners, which are comparative fit suppers to the MRE. The morning after appearance in Andar, the Afghan Army warriors grumbled about being ravenous, and the battle counselors expected to get them food from the nearby eateries. We discovered that the Afghan Army warriors didn't care for the Halal dinners, so they tossed the cases out of the rear of the pickups on the caravan with the assumption that the battle counselors would get more food. We didn't have any subsidizing and right now had given the instances of suppers. The show raised as the Afghan Army officers grumbled to the Afghan Army commanders that the battle consultants weren't supporting them.

The main opportunity I verged on performing emergency treatment happened on one evening on the Andar mission. Glidden felt exceptionally sick, and we figured it very well may be because of parchedness. I proposed to embed an intravenous line to give him a pack of saline. I pulled the clinical pack from behind the driver's seat and begun to acquire the clinical supplies when Glidden regurgitated. This second was about the very time that the doctor from Task Force Catamount stopped by our position, and he saw Glidden upchuck red and turned out to be extremely worried about regurgitating blood. Glidden had some red Gatorade before he retched, so he wasn't regurgitating blood. I didn't start an intravenous line, and I didn't need to utilize any emergency treatment abilities on the sending.

n September sixteenth, every one of the components combined on Miri to build up designated spots and security around the area place. The region community had its fantastic opening on September seventeenth, which acquired every one of the nearby older folks, the initiative of Task Force Catamount, and the 203rd Afghan Army Corps administration who showed up with their guides in a Blackhawk helicopter. We needed to give security from the helicopter arrival zone to the area community, yet I had the option to momentarily see the Wisconsin guide pioneers. Team Catamount had close air support from A-10 Thunderbolt "Warthog." The pilot directed a few extremely low flybys. The help we got from the A-10 made me one-sided in the A-10 versus the F-35 covertness airplane political fight.

A specialist sergeant counsel came to supplant Glidden and Weist. We put in a few days at the designated spots around Miri and were extremely dull days. The specialist sergeant guide and I split tasks. I wound up on a few more expanded watches with Obie the following several days, including one got off watch for in excess of seven miles somewhat in a residue storm. I

was at last supplanted on the tenth day, exceptionally prepared to get back to Sharana to rest and clean up.

KING OF BATTLE

"Remember your canines of war, your serious weapons, which are the most-to-be regarded contentions of the freedoms of rulers." –
Frederick the Great

I enjoyed and excelled in artillery fire direction and gunnery and continued with artillery assignments as a fire direction officer. I was the last assigned brigade fire control officer before the unit transformed. During my 27 long periods of administration, doing ordnance estimations and tackling gunnery issues was the most agreeable movement. I appreciated being a basic individual from a fundamental group to team up on explicit information from various sources to decide exact impacts with graphs, plain information, and robotization abilities. The discharge heading focus is viewed as the cerebrums of the field big guns group, with eyewitnesses incorporated with move units mentioning cannons and heavy armament specialists utilizing beast power to move 95-pound adjusts and applying exact settings on the big guns pieces.

The field manual for US Army mounted guns gunnery has in excess of 700 pages of definite guidelines on ballistics, shooting diagrams, shooting tables, and meteorological data, alongside directions for wellbeing and exceptional weapons to decide information. The cannons group's base components are the onlooker going about as the eyes and ears to find targets and afterward demand ordnance support from the mounted guns unit. The discharge heading focus gets the solicitation for ordnance and cycles strategic and specialized estimations to give to the mounted guns heavy weapons specialists. After the gunnery heavy weapons specialists discharge the round, the spectator will call the shoot heading focus again with adjustments. This cycle proceeds until the objective is obliterated, killed, or stifled per the move unit's requirements.

Necessary ordnance computations are the distance and bearing from the howitzer cannons to the objective to know what heading and point the cylinder needs to point, and how much powder to add to have the 95 pound round sway miles away. Mounted guns is a region weapon, implying that the round doesn't have to have an immediate hit on the objective, however needs to affect inside 50 yards of the objective to accomplish impacts. Notwithstanding, computations past the distance and reach are needed to accomplish most extreme outcomes rapidly. Estimation factors that influence the precision of an ordnance round incorporate howitzer height, target rise, powder temperature, wind speed, wind heading, air thickness, temperature, and surprisingly the world's pivot. I had an incredible feeling of achievement, doing mounted guns estimations to accomplish most extreme impacts with time criticalness. Current US mounted guns utilizes ruggedized PC frameworks to process these computations inside seconds.

All of the field cannons support in Afghanistan started from alliance powers, and there was distinct fascination with having the Afghan Army have the option to expect their discharge support. The Afghan Army big guns fighters got restricted big guns preparing for direct-shoot during their underlying preparing. There was tension from Combined Forces Command – Afghanistan level to have the Afghan Army big guns fighters fire the D-30 by implication. Our unit group pioneer said that Ressler and I were to make it happen.

two or three days after I got back from the Andar mission, my center changed from infantry backing to handle big guns support. The Afghan Army cannons official, Obie, and I flew from Sharana Provincial Reconstruction Team to Camp Phoenix to go to the principal Afghan Army big guns gathering. The motivation behind the three-day meeting at the Kabul Military Training Center was to unite Afghan Army cannons pioneers and ordnance battle counsels to build up the situation with all the gunnery organizations and direct examples. The Afghan Army likewise had a live-discharge showing with a few direct-shoot D-30 howitzers.

The ordnance meeting was intriguing, and there was a conversation on the most proficient method to lead Russian gunnery as their cycle is essentially not the same as the US. The Russian strategy utilizes 6,000 mils all around, and the US utilizes 6,400 mils all around. A mil is a unit of estimation more modest than a degree all around. Precise long-range gunnery discharge require point by point estimations. Moreover, the sights on the howitzer were unique, and there wasn't any preparation for eyewitnesses. Ressler and I would have a tremendous test sorting out the mechanical contrasts and how to utilize roundabout fires

safely.

essler had the option to start restricted gunnery preparing while I was on my leave toward the finish of July, and the Afghan Army ordnance discharged their D-30s direct-shoot into a cavern not very far outside of the base. Subsequent to getting back from leave toward the start of August, we went through around four days chipping away at pointing circles, terminating tables, and team drills before I was re-entrusted into infantry missions once more. Ressler and I struggled acquiring duplicates of guidance manuals and terminating tables, and a portion of the materials that we got were deficient and in Russian. In September 2006, the Afghan Army cannons organization got five additional D-30s and the fire bearing unit, a vital part to fire indirectly.

barely seven days after the mounted guns gathering, on October eleventh, Ressler, Obie, and I moved two D-30s, loads of ammo, and 15 Afghan Army ordnance troopers to Shkin. The arrangement was to incorporate into the Task Force Wolfpack areas to fire by implication. Nonetheless, we immediately ran into a few huge issues that would forestall this goal. The main obstruction was the freedom of flames as we were unable to guarantee cordial soldiers were not nearby as a significant number of the Special Forces missions were characterized. Moreover, the D-30 had range restricts that significantly decreased our accessible regions to target. We just put in a couple of days at Shkin before we were coordinated to move north to Bermel.

he troopers at Bermel were not anticipating us, so we were transient status. The battle guide group at Bermel was another Marine group, and they dwelled in the battle counsel's substantial structure. Ressler and I dozed on bunks in a B-Hut. The Marine battle counselor group boss said that we should seek shelter in their structure during rocket assaults as our pressed wood building would offer no insurance, and the dugouts were full. We left our firearm truck in the battle counselor leaving region nearby the Marine battle consultant building.

orking with the Task Force Catamount fire support official, I chose a point on a mountain, scope of roughly eight miles away close to the Pakistan line that had been a past rocket starting place, and could undoubtedly see with the JLENS. The Task Force Catamount fire support official, Task Force Catamount organization commandant and I had a worry about the Afghan Army ordnance as there was very little trust in the Afghan Army specialized information and guaranteeing the leeway of flames. One of the D-30s was seriously harmed during transportation making it non-functional. The unpleasant territory harmed the other D-30, however Ressler was able

to work with the Task Force Catamount upkeep area at Bermel to fix it enough to work.

Besides the rocket assaults, we went through the initial four days at Bermel evaluating and fixing the D-30s, planning with Task Force Catamount fire support official for leeway of flames, and going through group drills. There was huge worry about the Afghan Army ordnance ammo. The Afghan Army had many high hazardous rounds on the rear of several freight trucks. There was a need to get the big guns adjusts in light of the fact that we didn't need them to stroll off and become future side of the road bombs. With the quantity of rocket assaults as of late, there was a significant potential for an arbitrary rocket affecting the freight truck loaded up with high explosives. Bermel didn't have any capacity choices, however the Marine group pioneer could uphold us by getting two steel trailers that we could cover and block. The D-30s were emplaced just outside of the principle border and could be gotten to through the back entryway, yet were completely uncovered and offered no cover.

Ressler and I made an extraordinary group as he had ability in the mechanical working of the howitzer and team drills, and I knew discharge heading and gunnery. Ressler worked with the Afghan Army sergeant and group, and I worked with the Afghan Army mounted guns official. The Afghan Army mounted guns official had the option to set up the discharging plotting board to decide heading yet didn't have a clue how to wrap up of the gunnery estimations. I had the option to utilize the discharging tables and data from the US shoot course focus to figure the gunnery estimations. The

Afghan Army cannons official would send the firearm orders on his Afghan Army radio to the Afghan Army ordnance sergeant. I would radio the controls to Ressler to guarantee they were applied correctly.

On October nineteenth, we at long last had a go-ahead to fire. The Afghan Army cannons official plotted the objective on the mountain on his shooting plotting board, and I determined the firearm orders for the Afghan Army gunnery official to send. Ressler chose to utilize an additional a long cord and left our firearm truck behind the D-30 to give cover in the event that the D-30 failed. I utilized the JLENS to notice the D-30 and the effect and recorded the whole fire mission. The primary Afghan Army roundabout fire, roughly eight miles away, happened at 10:59 am Greenwich Mean Time on October nineteenth, 2006.

the D-30 terminating was significantly stronger than the US field cannons. The Task Force Catamount fire support official and I didn't notice the

sway yet thought we saw smoke right over the ridgeline and chose to rehash the fire mission to affirm. We didn't see the subsequent effect yet saw smoke in a similar area. I made a gunnery amendment, and we noticed the third round affecting inside 50 yards of the objective point. We called for three additional rounds and saw all rounds affecting around the objective. Ressler and I utilized a couple of the shell housings to make a "much obliged" gift to Task Force Catamount discharge support official and friends officer. We took pictures, and I utilized the JLENS recording to make a brief video. Team Catamount mounted the canister and photographs on the divider in the feasting office. Ressler and I chose to compose a short article for the Field Artillery Journal, an expert distribution at the US Army field gunnery central command. Our report, First to Fire, was distributed in the January-February 2007 version of the Field Artillery Journal.

I invested some energy that late evening auditing why we were askew on our underlying rounds. There are five prerequisites for precise shoot: target area, discharging unit area, weapon data, meteorological data, and computational systems. I was positive about the objective area with the utilization of the JLENS, and I was happy with the terminating unit area with the utilization of GPS. Force temperature and gag speed varieties wouldn't have huge contacts with range. The fundamental necessity that would influence the aftereffect of the rounds affecting long would be the meteorological data. In auditing the terminating, not set in stone that I wanted a reach revision for the pneumatic force. Since our base elevation was around 7,500 feet, and the round would go north of 8,000 feet over this, the pneumatic force at 15,000 feet would be lower, causing the round to go further. This computation would clarify why our initial two rounds affected over the ridgeline. The following day, with the air thickness data that I got from Task Force Wolfpack's fire course focus, we terminated four last adjusts at two unique targets and all round affected close the targets.

On the morning of October 22nd, the Task Force Catamount organization officer informed me that General Wardak, the Afghanistan Minister of Defense, and Lieutenant General Eikenberry would be traveling to Bermel later. They needed to perceive our endeavors and the endeavors of the occupant Afghan Army infantry brigade who had achievement in a firefight on October seventeenth with an expected 25 foe causalities. The Task Force Catamount organization leader proposed having a fire mission prepared to give a live-fire exhibition, so we went through the early daytime getting ready to fire. General Wardak

and Lieutenant General Eikenberry showed up by means of Blackhawks helicopters, Apaches helicopters, and Afghan Army helicopters, alongside a little escort that incorporated the 203rd Afghan Army Corps Commander and his consultant. The Afghan Army helicopters remained on the arrival zone and shut down while the rest left. The company went to the Afghan Army infantry force region first and apparently got cash bonuses.

While the escort was with the Afghan Army infantry brigade, we understood that the Afghan Army helicopters were straightforwardly online to the objective. We wouldn't have the option to direct the live-fire show. Since the visit time was restricted, we chose to do a dry fire mission exhibit. After the show, Lieutenant General Eikenberry distributed his test coins to the Afghan Army group, Ressler and I. By and large, administrators perceive extraordinary accomplishment with an effect grant of a little emblem bearing the association's insignia. There are currently many test currencies as units and associations have their plans, and they turned into an assortment of an exchanging thing. A test coin is an individual token and not perceived in faculty records. In any case, Lieutenant General Eikenberry's test coin from Combined Forces Command – Afghanistan is my most pined for grant or acknowledgment that I have gotten in my tactical profession. After certain photos and short conversations, the Blackhawk helicopters returned, and they all departed.

Immediately after the remainder of the helicopters left, we went under another rocket assault. The Afghan Army gunnery official and I were at that point went to the activities community to lead the live-shoot mission and ran the last couple of yards to get secret. When we got into the room, the Task Force Catamount fire support official inquired as to whether we were prepared to fire for a counter-fire mission. Since we were ready to lead the live-fire exhibition, everything was accessible. The Afghan Army ordnance official immediately plotted the matrix for the beginning of the rockets got from the radar. I processed the gunnery and weapon orders, and the Afghan Army ordnance official called the controls to the group. We terminated six rounds before the Task Force Catamount fire support official had us quit terminating as the Apache helicopters were back in the area.

I discovered a little while later that this counter-fire mission brought about ten causalities. As far as anyone knows, the Apache helicopters radioed the fight harm appraisal to the tasks community after they showed up back nearby. As I determined the gunnery piece of the mission, I played a huge part that

brought about those setbacks. Be that as it may, I don't have fortunate or unfortunate passionate sentiments as I was an individual from the group, we were a huge span away, I didn't see the harm, and I couldn't say whether the setbacks were injured or killed. In any case, it is great to realize that I could utilize my field big guns abilities in battle that had results.

For the following week at Bermel, the Afghan Army did nothing in light of a strict festival, and we didn't have a freedom of shoot. Team Wolfpack was shy of faculty, and I helped man one of their howitzers, including terminating. The M119A2 howitzer is a 105mm towed howitzer requires a group of somewhere around five warriors to fire three 30-pound adjusts each moment up to
10.9 miles. Team Wolfpack had a couple of fixed howitzers all things considered of the bases in eastern Afghanistan. I would have gotten a kick out of the chance to help more, yet I wasn't living with the Task Force Wolfpack and wouldn't be quickly accessible for counter-fire missions, so I just helped with a couple preplanned missions. A media team from CNN, Jennifer Eccleston, a cameraman, and a maker moved into our B-Hut for five days to ride alongside the Task Force Catamount components. Ressler and I helped the team in responding to inquiries regarding the region and terms. We persuaded them to incorporate our Afghan Army big guns officers into their story, which circulated on CNN Newsroom in November 9th.

The unit group pioneer at first let Ressler and I know that we would be at Bermel for two or three weeks. There were a lot of deferrals and changes to this arrangement. Administration at long last concluded that I would be reassigned to another situation in Gardez as the 203rd Afghan Army Corps Fire Support Coordinator and Ressler would remain in Bermel and train the following revolution of Afghan Army officers. The reassignment was essential for our Wisconsin counsel pioneer's arrangement to solidify the Wisconsin counselor group. I wasn't excessively amped up for returning to Gardez; be that as it may, the antagonistic mental impacts from the various rocket assaults were getting to me, and I was unable to stand by to move away from Bermel. On November fourth, a Blackhawk helicopter showed up to get me and take me to Gardez. I was the main traveler, and it was rare to be a sole traveler. I had the option to tune in on a portion of the discussions with the headset. I got some conversation with the Apache helicopter escort that said something regarding conceivable gag streaks. The Apache pilot showed he killed the objective. We flew over the whale territory highlight from Operation Anaconda, which was somewhat cool to see.

FREEDOM BIRD

"Getting back home from desolate spots, we all go somewhat frantic: regardless of whether from extraordinary individual achievement, or simply a the entire night drive, we are the last ones standing of a world no other person has at any point seen."

-

John Le Carre

Almost all of the Wisconsin advisor team had at least two assignments. The Wisconsin advisor team was initially assigned to the 205th Afghan Army Corps in Kandahar transferred to the 203rd Afghan Army Corps in July. With steady pivots of staff and evolving prerequisites, it was hard to monitor everybody. No one in Gardez was anticipating me, and I didn't have an assigned bunk, work area, or anyplace to go. I had my backpack from my central goal at Bermel, yet the remainder of my stuff was in Sharana, which I would get on a future caravan. I observed an unfilled bunk yet wound up moving B-Huts a few times before they set up a Wisconsin B-Hut.

The fire support facilitator was another position, and I didn't have a rundown of obligations and obligations. I needed to find a working environment of somebody who was gone and afterward move again when they returned and track down another work environment. One of my obligations was to assist with organizing a Mongolian group between Camp Phoenix and our two detachments. Mongolia sent around twelve troopers who were D-30 specialists and had the legitimate apparatuses and gear to support the D-30s. They were booked to go to every one of the five corps regions to keep up with every one of the howitzers, and I needed to arrange the two detachments getting their D-30s to Gardez and having a space accessible for the Mongolian group to work. Notwithstanding the Mongolian group coordination, I should guide the senior Afghan Army mounted guns official on the corps staff. In any case, I didn't have a mediator, and the Afghan Army cannons official was gone very often.

For Thanksgiving in Gardez, project workers made game plans to have a rotisserie turkey and stove cooked turkey. Customarily, officials serve occasion suppers, and I helped serve the stove simmered turkey. This occasion was the main significant occasion that I spent away from my family. The feast was nice yet appeared to be a ho-murmur day.

My four-day pass in November was postponed and rescheduled for mid-December. Notwithstanding our fourteen day leave, we could have the chance to get a four-day pass to Qatar yet was subject to mission, rank, plans, so not every person got a pass. Getting a pass would be an incredible chance to move away for a couple of days and partake in a brew in a warm climate. I passed on Gardez to Camp Phoenix on 7:30 am on December fourth. Our little escort went through Sharana and Ghazni, and, with weighty snow, we didn't show up in Camp Phoenix until 7:00 pm. I was fortunate to be a driver and get a portion of the weapon truck warmer's advantages as our heavy armament specialist immediately turned into a snow-shrouded Popsicle. Following a couple of long periods of wonderful transient status, our stream freight plane took off from Bagram to Qatar. The day of appearance doesn't consider a spend day, and we showed up soon after 12 PM; subsequently, after our briefings and a short rest, we had very nearly a full extra day.

Unfortunately, because of photograph limitations, I don't have any photographs of my take a break. I connected up with two battle guides from different units. We just connected up at supper and for bar time, and we did whatever we might feel like doing during the day. Qatar was radiant and warm, and I had the option to wear shorts and a polo shirt. The base was fanned out, and gigantic stockrooms contained everything. The dozing quarters were 12-man rooms with lofts, and the lights remained off on the grounds that faculty were going back and forth during all hours, every hours. The feasting office was around a 15-minute walk, however it was awesome as it was by a long shot the best food during the entire organization. They had genuine plates and tableware and even had dessert coolers and Baskin Robbins frozen yogurt. It was around a five-minute stroll from our dozing quarters to the spirit building, which contained a PC lab, game rooms, computer game control center, and a bar region in the back. You were restricted to three beverages and needed to filter your recognizable proof card when you bought the $5 cocktails.

You could take a van transport to the shoppette and the Chili's café. I went to the shoppette the primary day and bought an excellent pearl neckband and hoops for my significant other We wound up eating at Chili's twice. During the day, I went to the PC lab for email and played a great deal of Halo and Grand Theft Auto video games.

On the third day of the pass, I had the option to pursue an outing. The assurance group had two visits accessible, one was a roadtrip to a shopping center, and the different was going to the ridges. There was some huge soccer competition nearby, so they dropped the shopping center outings for the week while I was in Qatar, however I had the option to pursue the ridges. The little gathering of us stacked up in two Land Cruisers SUVs and drove close to the base. They pulled off the street into the huge ridges and collapsed their tires for better foothold. We cruised all over for some time and afterward halted at a little tent retreat region on the Persian Gulf. We had a grill lunch, played sand volleyball, and swam in the Persian Gulf. Despite the fact that I didn't know anybody in our gathering, I made some pleasant memories. At the point when we drove out of the rises, we halted at the corner store to blow up the tires and got back to the base. Because of troop decreases in the theater, the spirit program shut in 2011.

We got an additional a spend day due to airplane accessibility and took a C-130 propeller freight airplane conveying a firearm truck from Qatar to Kabul. I was in transient status at Camp Phoenix for a couple of days, hanging tight for a ride back to Gardez. The USO/Sergeant Major of the Army visit had a show at Camp Phoenix while I was there, and I had the option to see the Dallas Cowboy team promoters, Al Franken, The Washington Projects, Keni Thomas, Leeann Tweeden, Mark Wills, and

Darryl Worley. It was a thrilling show, however it was cold outside. I don't figure my feet could be any more frozen, and it hurt to stroll back to my tent. I was the heavy armament specialist in a 5-ton truck on the caravan back to Gardez on December 23rd and had 12 bundles hanging tight for me on my bunk. I chose to delay until Christmas morning to open them. As an extraordinary Christmas present, we got several creeps of snow on Christmas Eve. I appreciated getting bundles while sent. Getting genuine letters and postcards is superb, and I kept all that I got yet wasn't required as we had restricted email. I'm particularly thankful to get bundles that contained Starbucks Double Shot Espresso jars of espresso and Jelly Belly Sport Beans. y significant other sent me a couple of helpful things consistently, for example, sheets and my favored body wash.

was the shoot support organizer in the name however was a unique undertakings official. I arranged a Saint Barbara big guns grant service on January sixth, which Ressler and my Afghan Army corps big guns official each got the Honorable Order of Saint Barbara grants. I managed the Field Artillery Association, and the function was facilitated by the ordnance detachment leader and the 203rd Afghan Army Corps Commanding General. The

translators deciphered the tale of Saint Barbara, punch bowl service, and grants show with around 50 US and Afghan Army personnel.

I composed a few bits of the Afghan Army corps order and staff practice intended to help the Afghan Army staff figure out together through various problems and issues. More than three days, the battle guide gave things to the corps staff to foster a game plan. A portion of the issues we created were: a transport rollover with mass setbacks, a side of the road bomb at a base entryway, or a base getting defiled water. I additionally planned a portion of our impending Wisconsin guide group's flight plans.

The Wisconsin counsel pioneers passed on mid-January to get back to Camp Shelby, MS, to brief forthcoming battle counselor revolutions about their encounters. Most days at Gardez was attempting to browse email some place and watching films and TV. The Wisconsin B-Hut had an Armed Forces Network association, and we had the option to get a TV. The show choice wasn't great, however it was something special to do. I delighted in watching Emeril Lagasse on his cooking show, which was on after supper. I didn't have an activities community or work area region to work and wound up watching a lot more films and Armed Forces Network. You would have rather not seem exhausted in light of the fact that you could get entrusted for certain inconsequential obligations, so I invested a ton of energy in the B-Hut. The colder time of year fatigue was more awful as we were drawing nearer to returning home, and we were stuck on a snow-shrouded base. There were days, particularly the most recent few months when my main notes on my schedule expressed that everything I did was browsed email and watched movies.

a few group on the base had little assortments of DVDs, however there was a ton of film sharing on outer hard drives. I wound up with just about 500 films on my outside hard drive. The packed film's quality is very feeble, and a portion of the motion pictures were bootleg market where somebody in the Far East would video record another film in the theater, and the neighborhood Afghans would sell these DVDs at the marketplaces. These films would be too difficult to even consider looking as the sound quality was second rate as it recorded individuals' discussions and chuckling, or the image was screwy. My Palm Pilot was very convenient to fill a portion of the vacations. My beloved games were Bejeweled, Drug Wars, and Solitaire. Since my Palm Pilot was little, I kept it in my pocket more often than not and could utilize it as a music player, and I monitored day by day features in the calendar.

Things were changing in my last month of arrangement. Lieutenant General Eikenberry left Combined Forces Command – Afghanistan and the association disbanded. Global Security Assistance Force was assuming control over the eastern space of Afghanistan. The guide center was moving from the Afghan Army to Afghan Police, and the Afghan Army was accepting our more established style weapon trucks and M16 rifles. This second was a fantastic opportunity to be going home as there was almost no certainty with the Afghan Police, and a large portion of the battle counsels would have rather not take on that job. There was worry about handling this hardware to the Afghan Army in view of their absence of support and responsibility, and the material had a higher danger of falling into the adversary's hands.

The circumstance of my arrangement settled with the battling season cycle. Regularly, battling and assaults drop altogether throughout the cold weather a very long time in eastern Afghanistan. The adversary is thought to pull out to Pakistan to refit. As spring shows up, the assaults gradually grow into the late spring battling season. We showed up in Afghanistan at the finish of February, which permitted us an opportunity to adapt to the rise that arrived at the midpoint of around 7,500 feet and get orientated with the association. My late spring months were feverish and had some mission consistently. The colder time of year season, being at Gardez and not having a genuine task, come about in huge downtime.

Before we left Gardez, the work force official gave me my Bronze Star Medal and authentication. I stashed it securely in my sacks. At that point, I absolutely needed to keep things moving and return home and was irritated by the unessential guidelines, however there was no declaration, arrangement, or service. As recently referenced, there were a great deal of embellishment, dramatization, and bits of gossip over grants. I felt like I got what I merited and didn't require uncommon acknowledgment. I gave my features in a record to my rater. The greater part of it was utilized in exactly the same words for my assessment and grant proposal as he didn't have direct information on what I had accomplished.

It was thrilling on the morning of February fifteenth as we got into the weapon trucks to caravan to Camp Phoenix and began our excursion home. I attempted to travel gently, so I transported a sack of hardware home toward the finish of January yet at the same time had a full duffle pack, full rucksack, body protection, and cap. I was a traveler in this caravan and was the possibly time all sending when I sat in the secondary lounge of a firearm truck. While in Camp Phoenix, we went through stations to plan to leave the theater, which included having Navy Customs staff go through the entirety of our duffle sacks prior to palletizing for delivery. At Bagram, we needed to go through Navy Customs again as they assessed our portable things and whatever else with the rest of our personal effects. We flew in a fly cargo

plane to Manas Air Force Base to authoritatively sign out of the venue following 363 days. We left the following day on a sanctioned business aircraft, normally alluded to as "opportunity bird," and showed up in Gulfport, MS on February 22nd with delays in Baku, Azerbaijan, Shannon, Ireland, and New York JFK. The Wisconsin counsel pioneers were sitting tight for us as we got off the plane, and we took a sanction transport to Camp Shelby. We were at Camp Shelby for grounding for under a day and a half, where we turned in our weapons, went through clinical screenings, and marked our DD Form 214, Certificate of Discharge.

We took a contract transport rather than a business trip to get back to Madison and was possibly for the best as there was a blizzard in Wisconsin when we showed up on February 24th. The transport was almost vacant as there were just 15 travelers for the whole transport, however it was all the while testing to settle in to endeavor rest. We halted at a Crackle Barrel eatery some place in Illinois to clean up and eat. My parents in law from Manitowoc,

Wisconsin, and brother by marriage's family from Wausau, Wisconsin, chosen not to drive with the climate conditions. We were delivered after an exceptionally short homecoming festivity with the state initiative on the express central command's drill floor. My family proceeded with the festival with lunch at Carlos O'kelly's, a Mexican café in Madison, and I partook in a margarita.

Ultimately, I am extremely appreciative that I am alive and wasn't harmed. Past a couple of risky circumstances, I settled on some helpless decisions. The main eye insurance I utilized was my residue goggles while gunning. I didn't wear my gave ballistic eye insurance. I had ear insurance on my body shield, however possibly utilized them when I was on an airplane. There were watches where I would eliminate my head protector and wear my cap while in the bring forth at a designated spot and didn't regularly wear my cap while driving.

I just started to expose the Afghan culture. I had lunch in a nearby eatery with the Marine battle counselors, was welcomed into a mud-walled Afghan home during a residue storm in Andar, looked through a couple of yards, and strolled by neighborhood shops. I ate naan, drank chai, attempted a few meats, and partook in the rice. Being a battle counsel permitted me to encounter the way of life more so than a standard soldier.

One of the normal subjects for battle troopers is fraternity and brotherhood, particularly during horrendous mishaps. With my remarkable arrangement experience and various tasks, I never fostered that exceptional bond with anybody. A significant number of my missions and undertakings were with different

individuals, and I am appreciative that I caught my encounters with notes, messages, and photographs to epitomize my own insight. I was associated with: 55 caravans, 32 watches, 21 rocket assaults, 12 base security power missions, four side of the road bomb assaults, three fast response power missions, two firefights, and one gentle instance of post-horrible pressure problem. I pulled the trigger on the M119A2 howitzer in light of the adversary, and I shot the short suppressive shoot on the medium automatic weapon because of the foe. I never shot my gun or rifle.

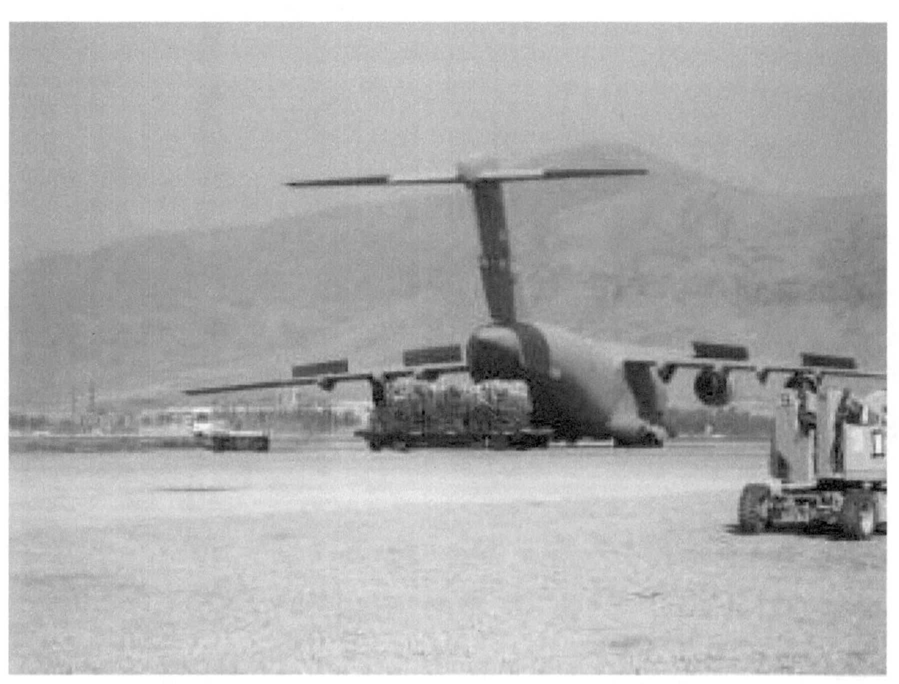

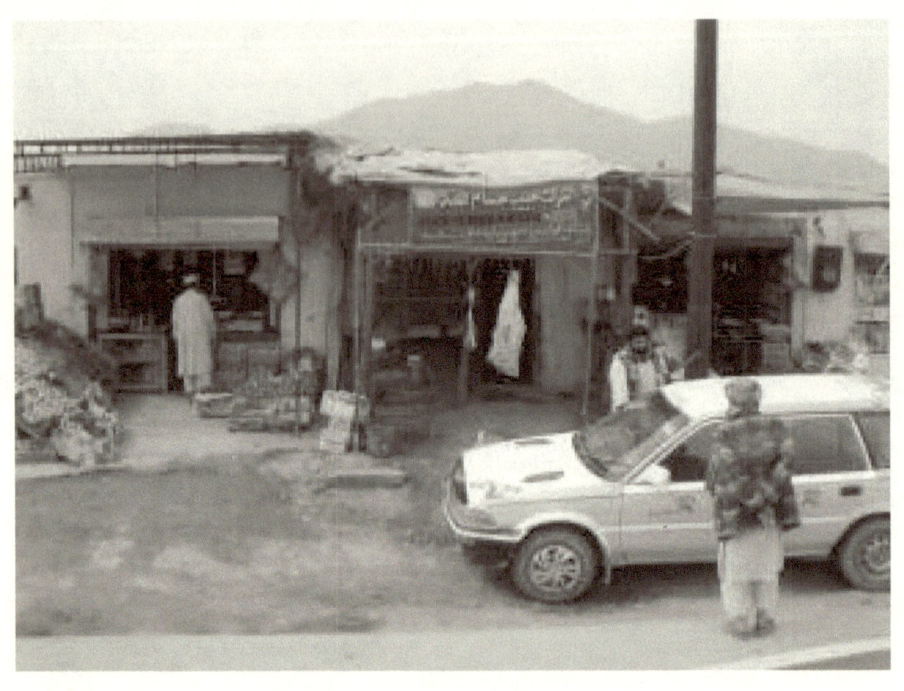

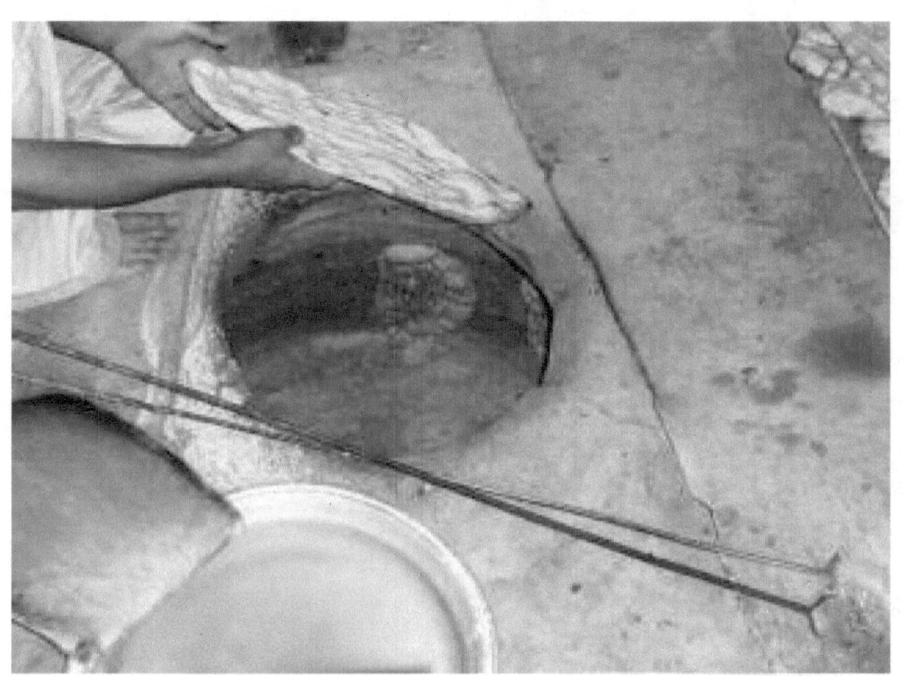

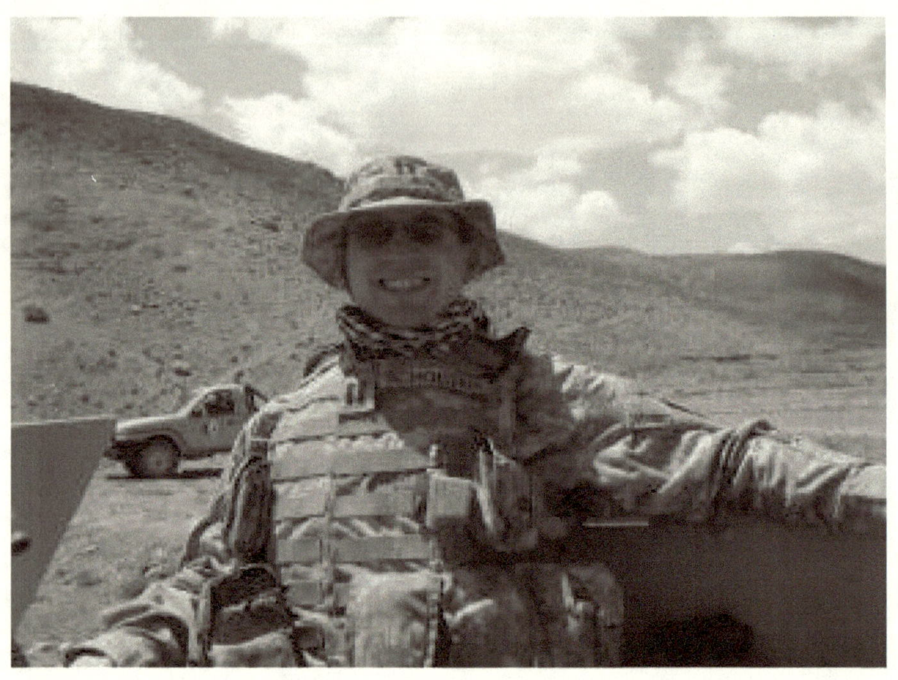

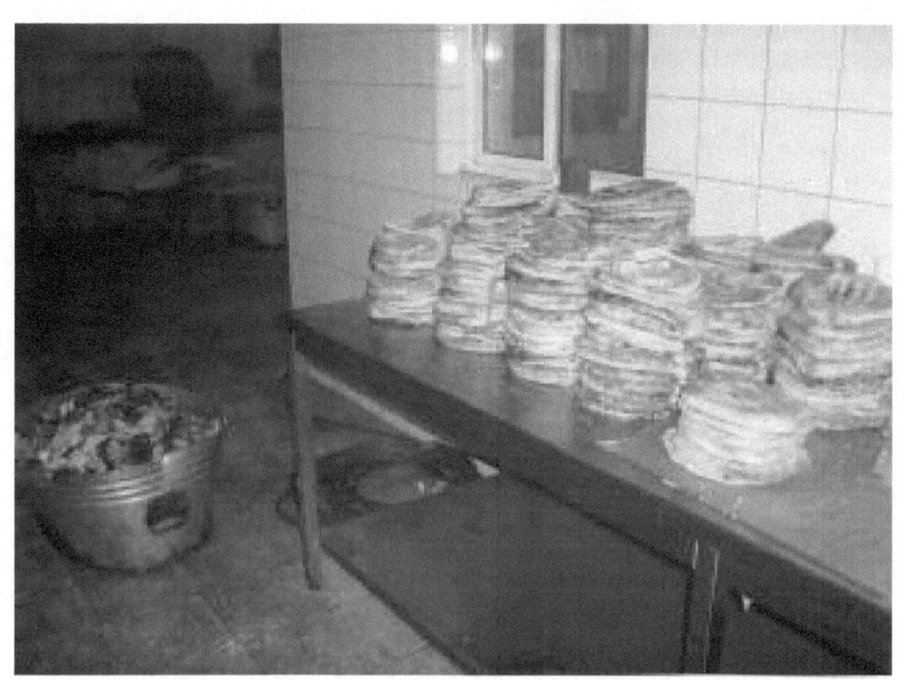

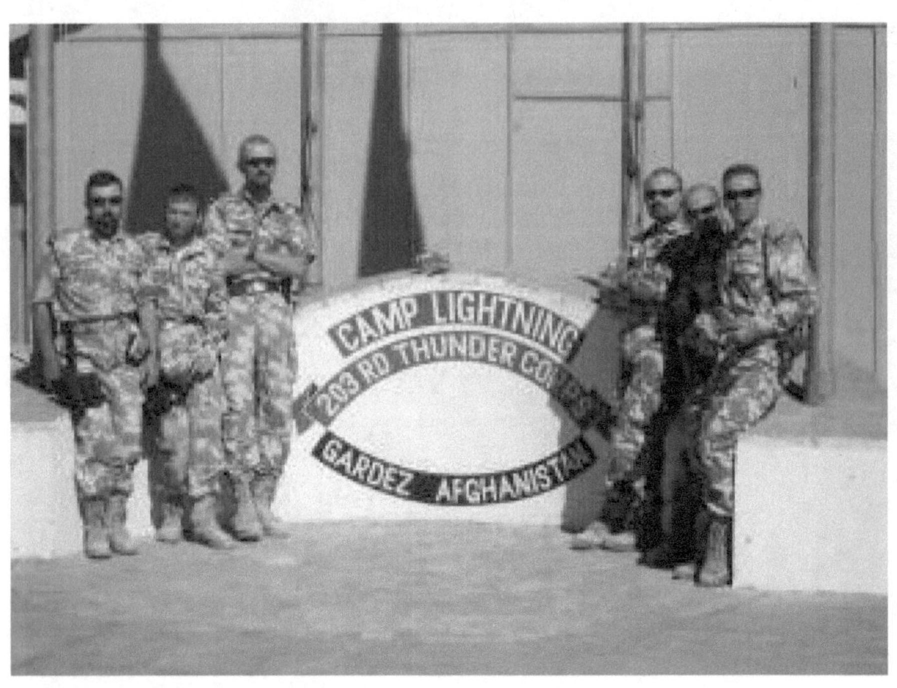
CAMP LIGHTNING
203 RD THUNDER CORPS
GARDEZ AFGHANISTAN

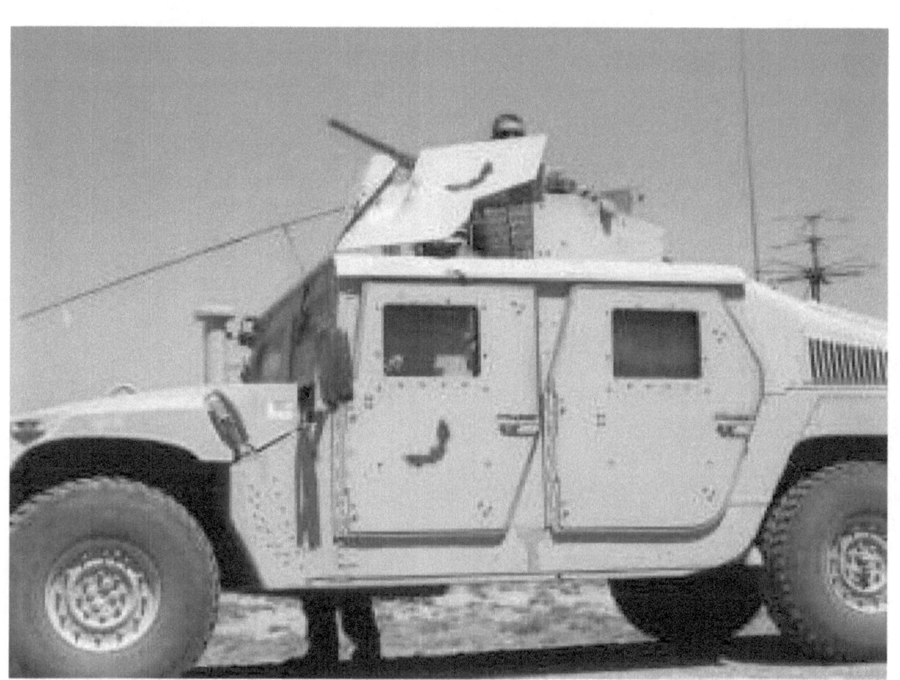

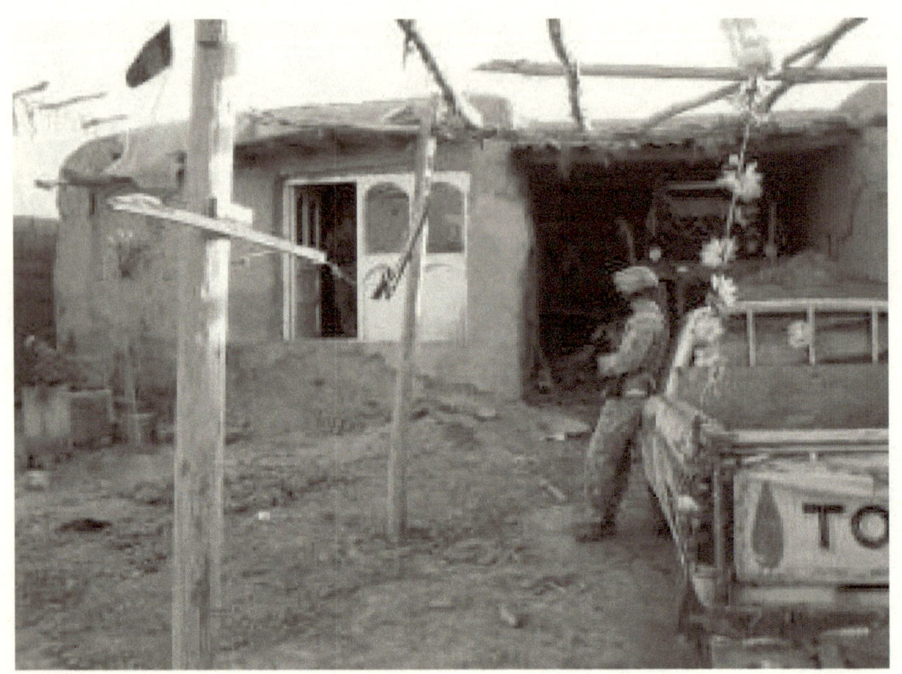
TO

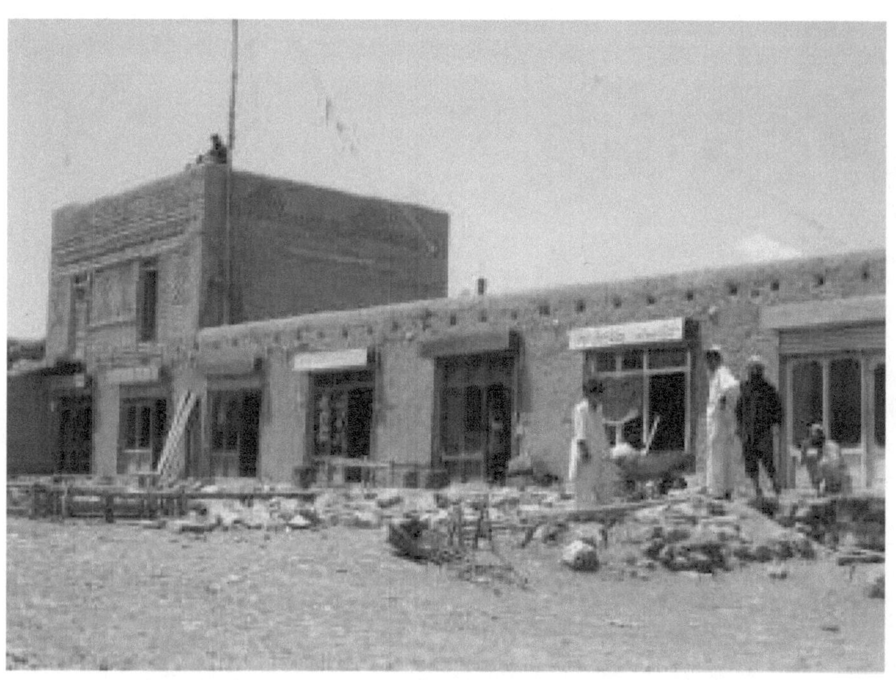

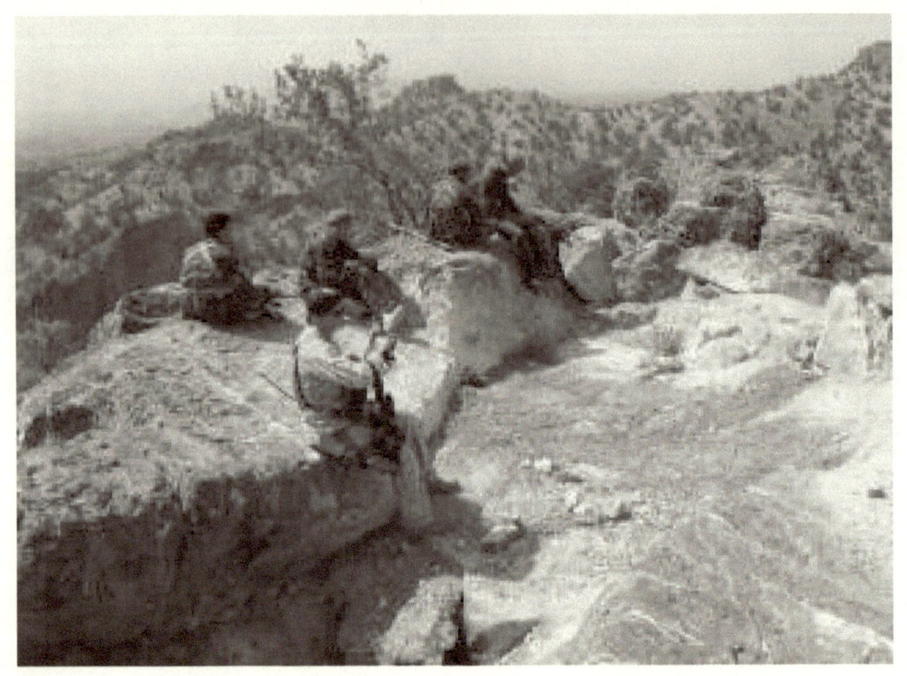

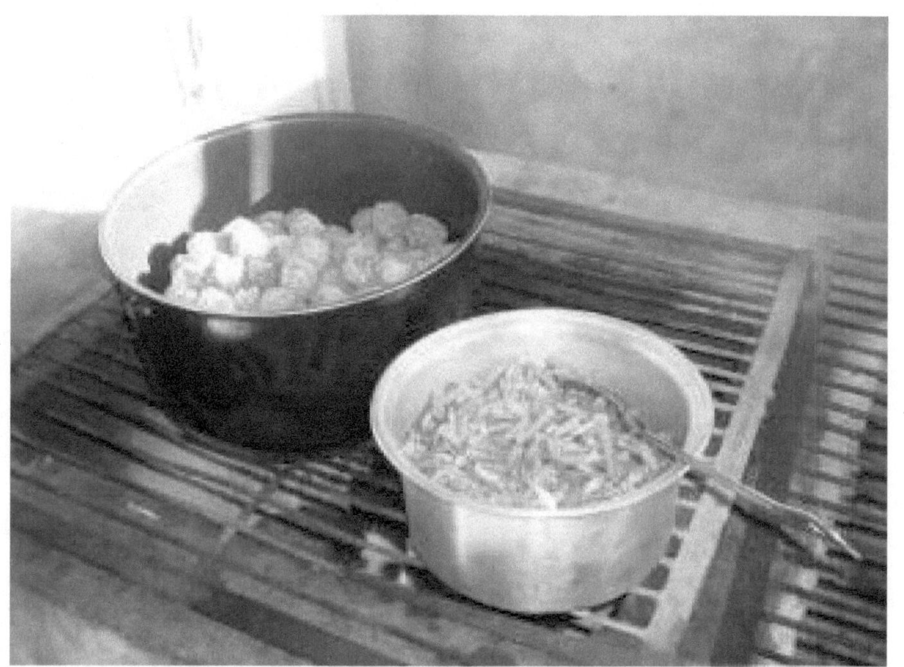

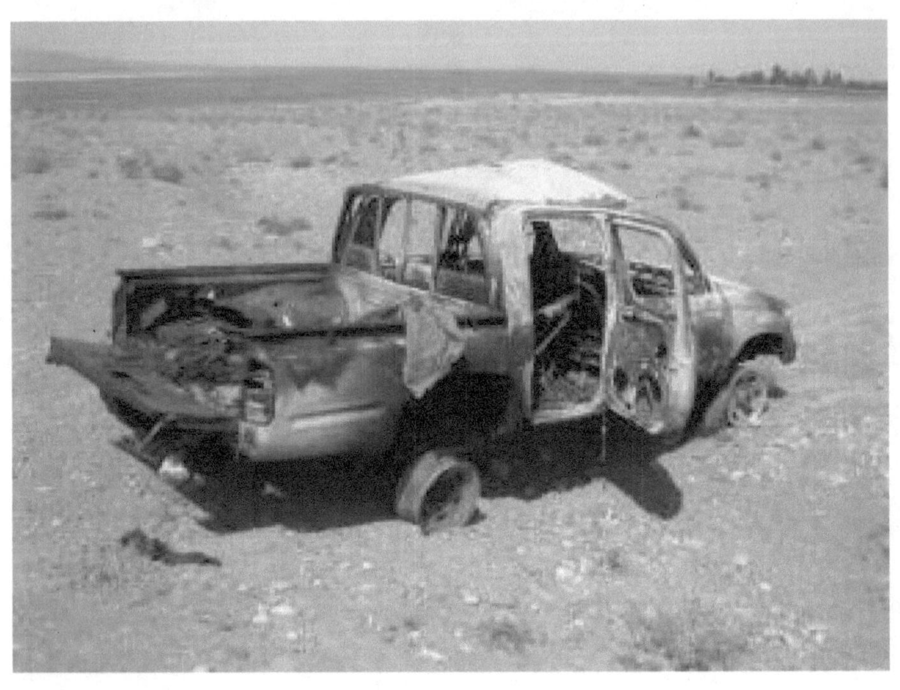

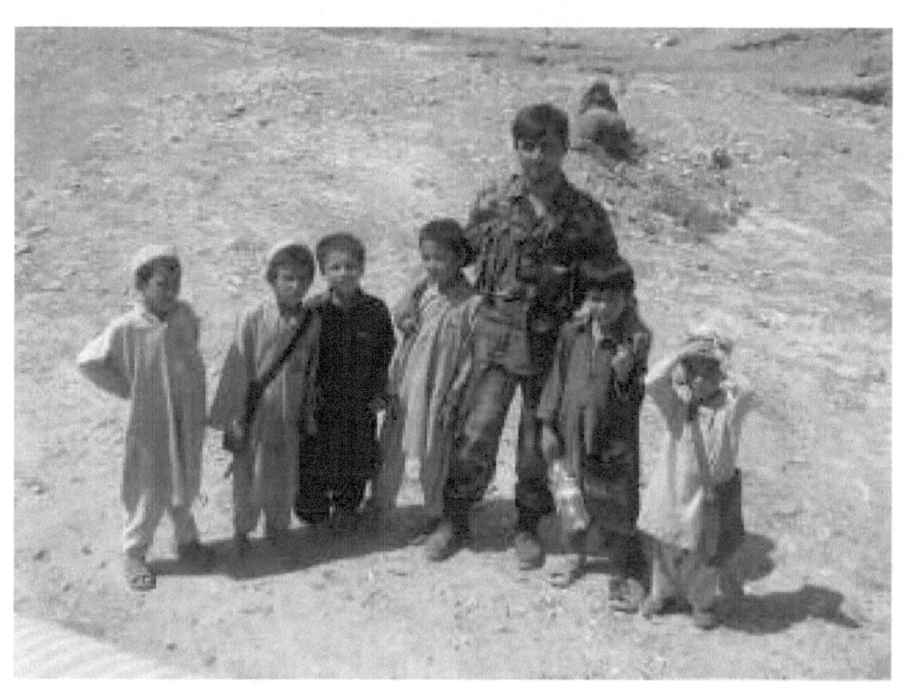

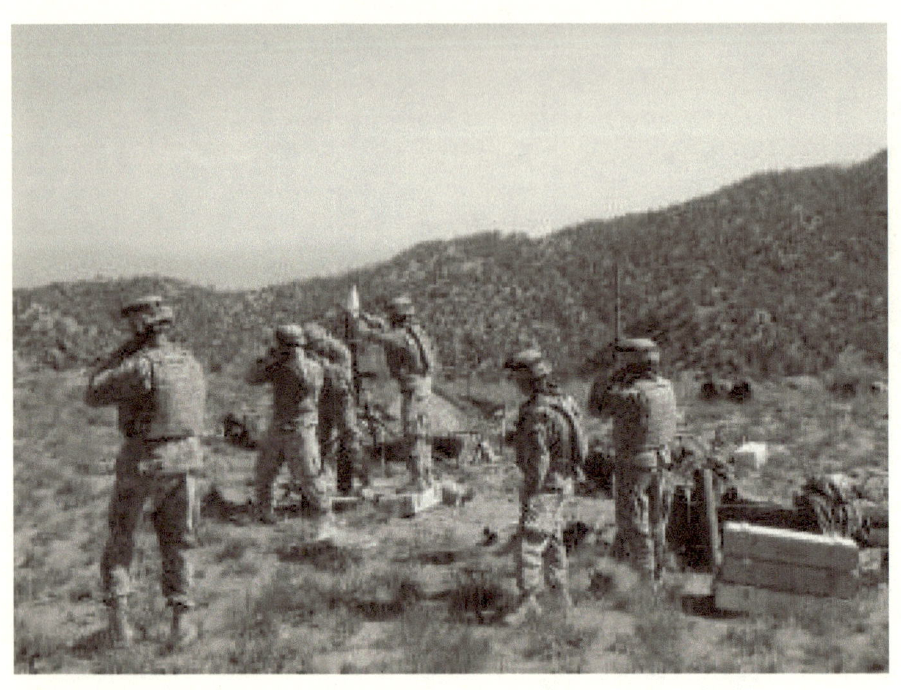

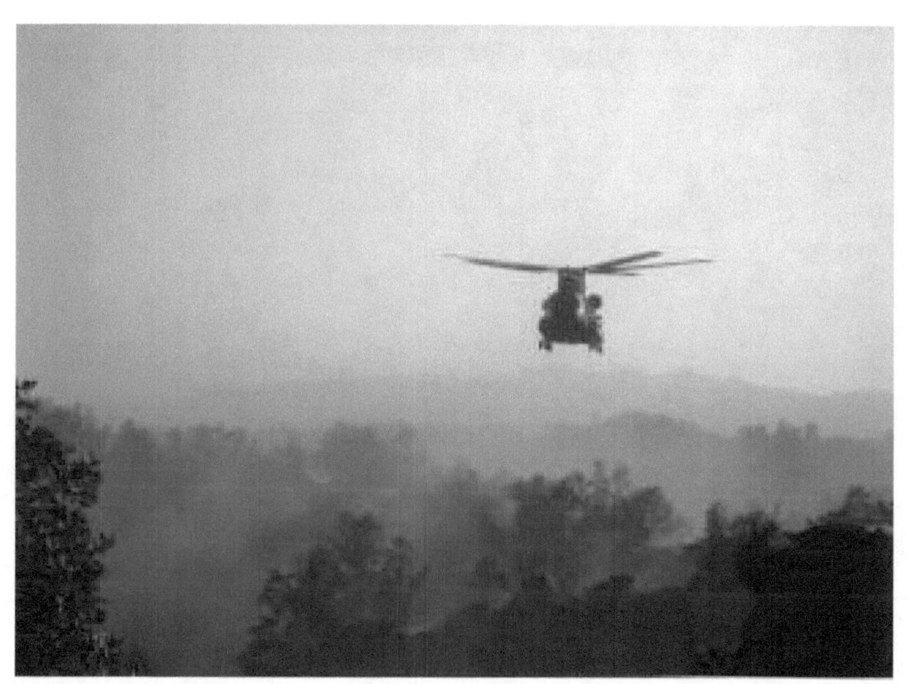

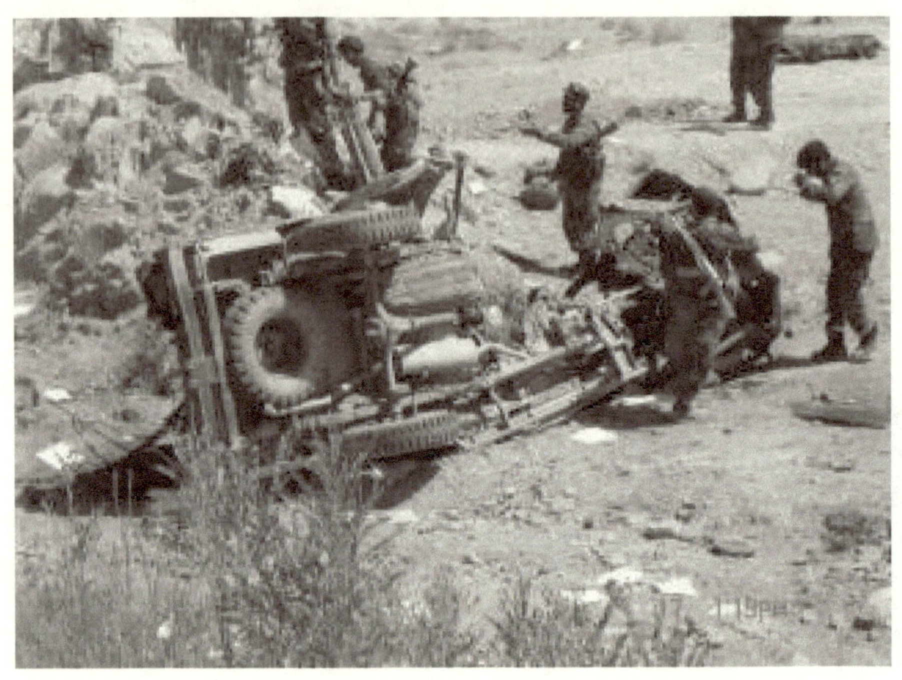

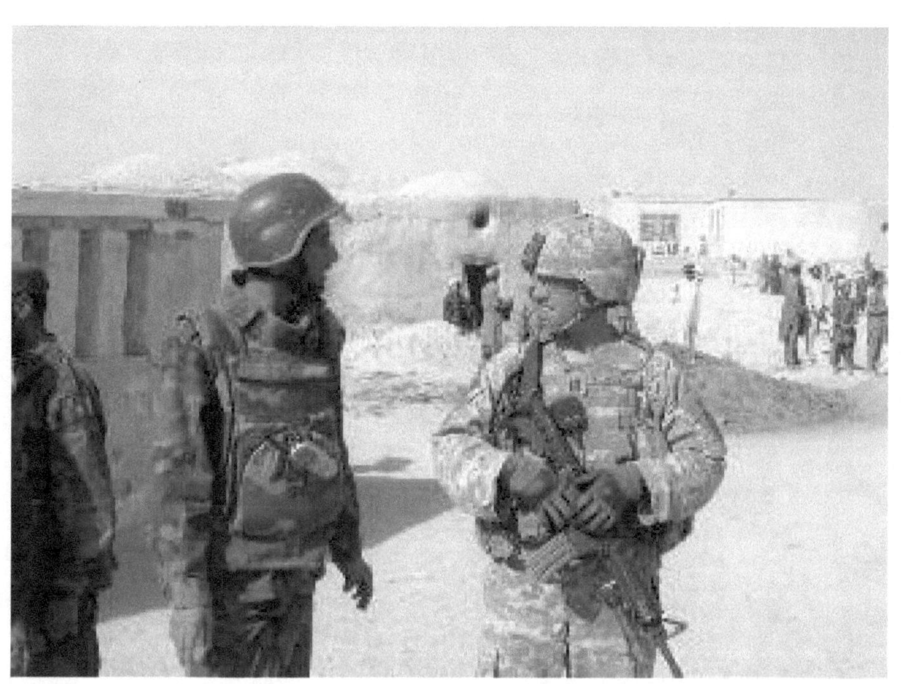

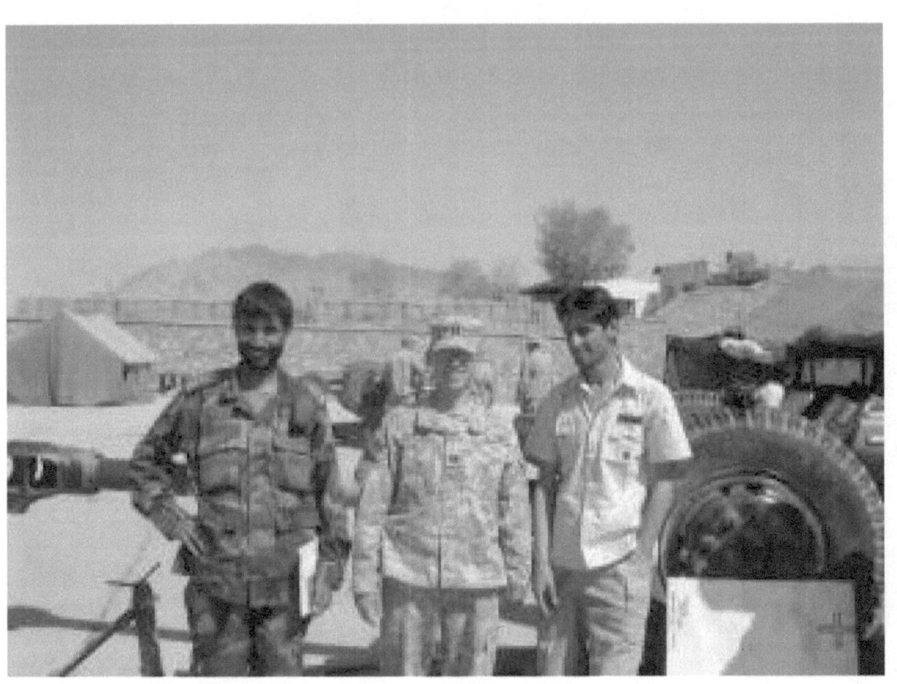

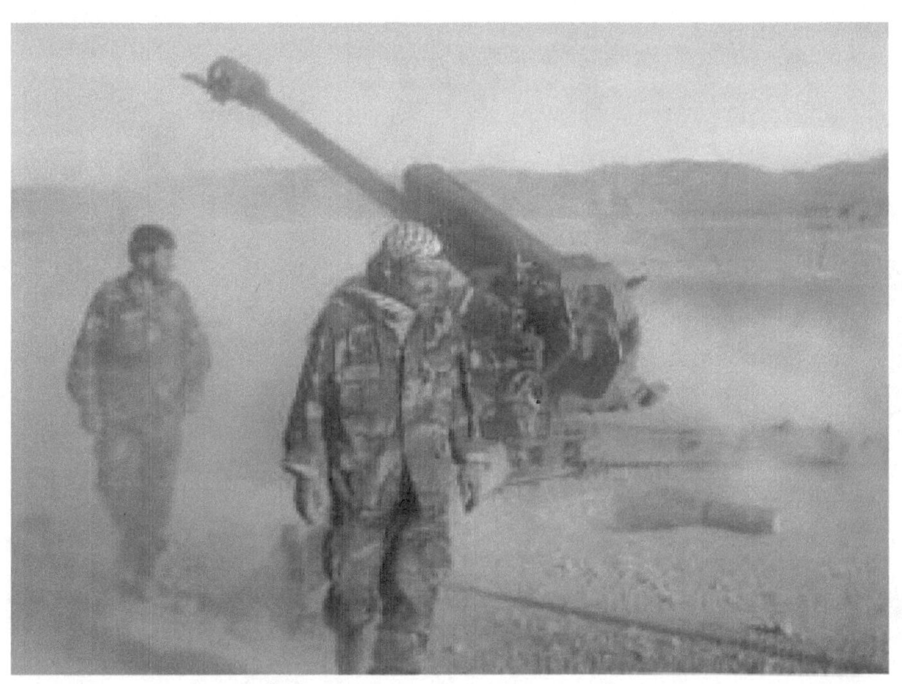

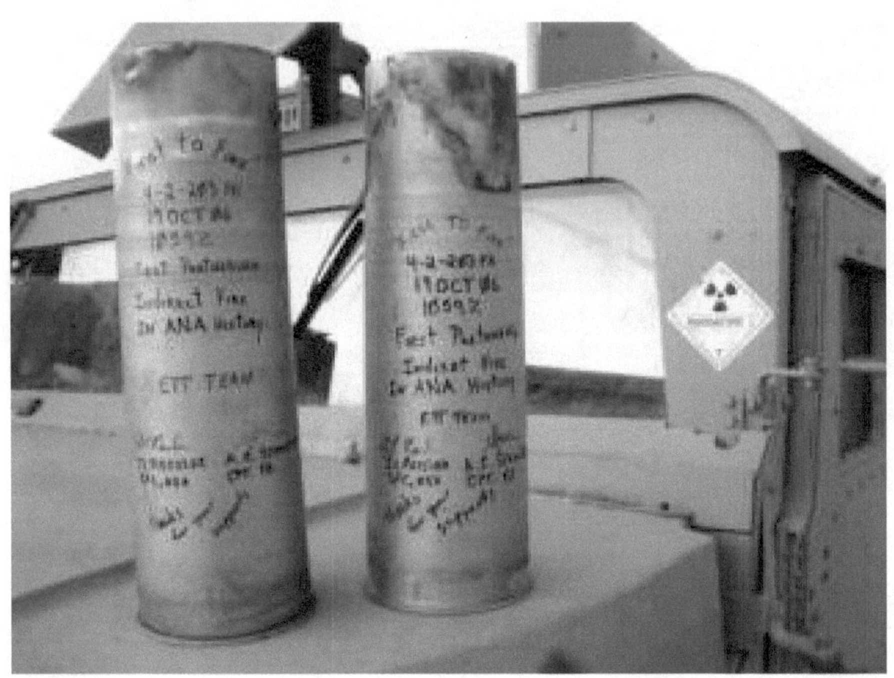
19 OCT 06
ETT TEAM

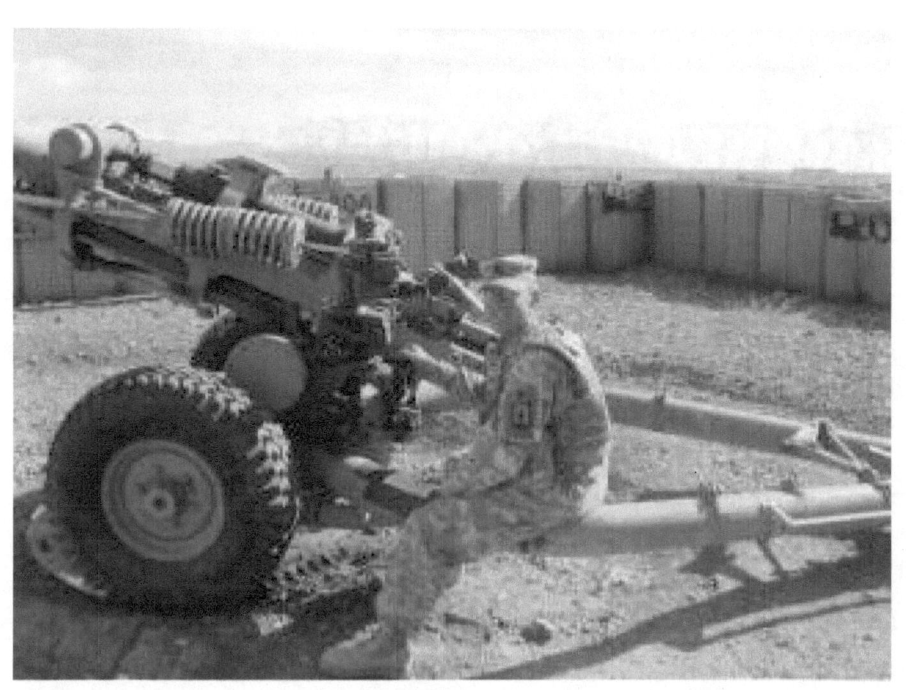

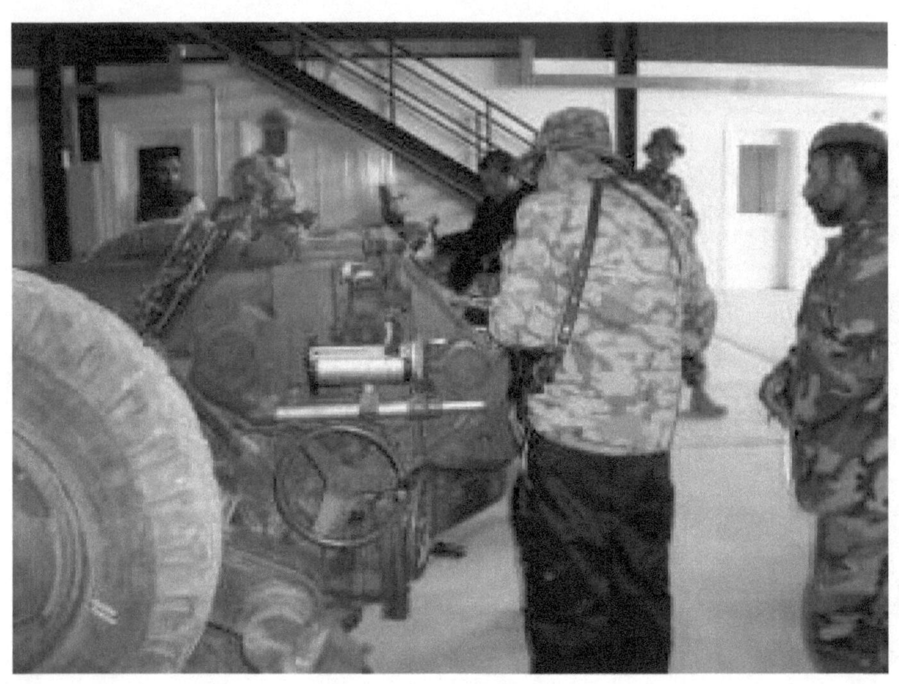

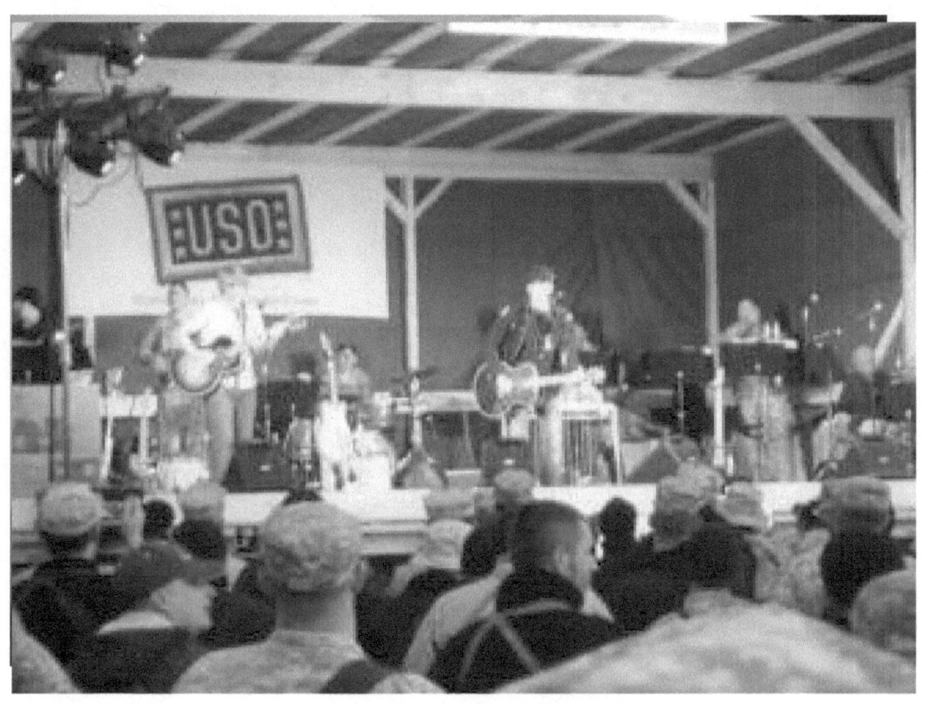
USO

PART TWO

POSTTRAUMATIC STRESS INJURIES

TRANSITION

"Don't pass judgment on individuals. You don't have the foggiest idea what sort of fight they are battling" - unknown

Approximately eight years after returning from Afghanistan, something emotionally was not quite right. I had low work engagement, my daughter became more independent, my marriage was comfortable, and I had no informal organizations. I had additional undesirable contemplations and pictures from the negative parts of my arrangement. I saw that my practices changed and adversely affected my work and public activity. I utilized withdrawal and evasion as ways of dealing with stress to the mark of separation. I depended on fanatical practices to give the solace of dependability. Understanding post-horrendous pressure injury was an extensive and testing process. A post-horrendous pressure injury happens at a point on schedule, however it has a wide range of manifestations and is marginally unique for everybody. It was hard for me to distinguish what the manifestations meant for me, and it was more difficult to request help because of the disgrace around post-horrendous pressure problem. I have a superior comprehension of post-horrendous pressure, what it has meant for me, and what helped me for the board for this imperceptible injury. I likewise became mindful of moral injury and how it varies from post-horrendous stress.

had one battle sending in my 27-year military profession. Upon redeployment, I felt that I was a superior military official on account of my remarkable encounters. Numerous incredible things occurred on my arrangement, such as working with far off countries and being a piece of a verifiable mounted guns mission. I got acknowledgment on my uniform for battle openness, similar to awards, patches, and the battle identification. In any case, a portion of the battle openness adjusted my feelings, sentiments, and changed my practices. It was practically eight

years after my organization when I found that I had post-horrible pressure problem (PTSD).

Like numerous others, I had the feeling that those experiencing their battle encounters seemed feeble or searching for a reason for awful conduct. In the same way as other others, I felt that those people with PTSD saw horrendous things and went to liquor, medications, viciousness, and self destruction. I envisioned that PTSD resembled a compound broke leg, where you could see the clear manifestations and acquire a standard treatment convention. I had no clue about that PTSD could be quick or deferred and vacillate with force. I'm not an extreme fighter, and numerous different officers had more serious and various organizations. I'm not an emotional wellness subject matter expert and see all parts of PTSD and its belongings. I do know what PTSD meant for me and my hypotheses on why.

t is fundamental to comprehend that PTSD isn't a major issue with somebody and that PTSD is something that happened to somebody. Previous President George W. Shrubbery expressed, "We're disposing of the D (in PTSD). PTS is a physical issue; it's anything but a turmoil. The issue is the point at which you consider it an issue, (veterans) don't figure they can be dealt with." In the most fundamental sense, PTSI is from an exceptionally awful accident that happened to somebody, and their mind doesn't completely handle the occasion. General (Ret) Peter Chiarelli, previous Vice Chief of Staff of the United States Army, upheld the previous President's comments by expressing, "It is a physical issue. Considering the condition a "jumble" propagates an inclination against the emotional well-being sickness and "has the undertone of being something a prior issue that an individual has" before they came into the Army and "causes the individual to appear to be frail." I am proceeding to break the shame; consequently, I will allude to the post-awful pressure condition as a physical issue, post-horrible pressure injury (PTSI).

he Governor of the State of Wisconsin broadcasted June 27th as Posttraumatic Stress Injury Awareness. Conversely, post-horrendous pressure wounds are crippling injuries to the mind, which can happen following openness to battle and other awful mishaps. In correlation, post-horrible pressure has generally been considered a psychological well-being disease brought about by a prior blemish in the singular's mind. The expression "Post-horrible Stress Disorder" conveys a disgrace that sustains this confusion. Gold country, Iowa, Arkansas, and other state Governors and legislatures have comparative decrees to reflect post-horrendous pressure as a physical issue. It required some investment to understand that something was off-base and converse with somebody, and a simple

name change would not have had an effect. Be that as it may, with an analysis, I can excuse a physical issue rather than an issue. It is more straightforward to acknowledge this condition as a physical issue as its start was at an awful, hazardous point on schedule. My PTSI indications gradually expanded over the long run, however the awful effect was a second on schedule.

I was organically impacted the evening of the base assault that affected my emotional well-being. I feel more calm, portraying how I was harmed instead of how I fostered a problem. The circumstance and occasions the evening of the base assault overpowered my mind's capacity to process everything and were naturally impacted. I didn't foster an issue; I caused a psychological well-being injury. There is a distinction between psychological wellness and conduct wellbeing, albeit many individuals utilize the terms conversely. Psychological well-being incorporates conditions that are acquired or include mind science, while conduct wellbeing centers around propensities. Emotional wellness conditions, like PTSI, may require diverse treatment programs than social medical issue, like betting or liquor addictions. It is pervasive for an individual to have co-happening problems, for example, a substance misuse issue and an emotional well-being disorder.

The Department of Veterans Affairs regulates the National Center for PTSD. The National Center for PTSD has the accompanying posted on their site (n.d. recovered from https://www.ptsd.va.gov):

PTSD side effects generally start before long the awful accident, however they may not show up until months or a long time later. They likewise may travel every which way over numerous years. There are four kinds of PTSD manifestations, however they may not be something similar for everybody. Every individual encounters manifestations in their way.

1. Reliving the occasion (likewise called re-encountering side effects). Recollections of the horrendous accident can return whenever. You might feel a similar dread and

2. Avoiding circumstances that help you to remember the occasion. You might attempt to keep away from circumstances or individuals that trigger recollections of the horrible event.

3. Negative changes in convictions and sentiments. The manner in which you contemplate yourself as well as other people changes on account of the injury. You might not have good or cherishing inclinations toward others and may avoid relationships.

4. Feeling keyed up (likewise called hyperarousal). You might be unsteady or consistently ready and keeping watch for risk. You may abruptly become

5.

6.

irate or crabby. This is referred to as hyperarousal.

PTSI is recognized as a mental condition and influences up to 3.5% of the US populace. In everyday terms, the mind processes an awful accident at a more profound level, yet it has not enough pre-arranged for the occasion. Since the recollections are at a more profound level, these horrendous recollections could be enduring, and the individual may not intentionally recognize triggers. PTSI additionally has actual impacts, disturbing the cerebrum synapses, and various indications can go from wretchedness, uneasiness, a reduction of confidence, expanded pulse, and numerous others.

PTSI can start very quickly, or it might advance throughout the long term or a long time and be gentle to totally incapacitating. PTSI likewise is frequently muddled by different problems, for example, liquor and illicit drug use, sadness, tension, outrage, and numerous different issues. It is hard to represent every one of those impacted by PTSI precisely. Screening upon redeployment might recognize a portion of the indications, yet the legitimate testing is subject to genuine revelation from the impacted trooper. Moreover, the screenings just measure a point on schedule and won't precisely represent postponed reactions.

Understanding and looking for help are the initial phases in getting therapy. There is no conclusive treatment or a normalized treatment convention, as emotional wellness is an intricate issue to explore and see completely. The most acknowledged PTSI treatment choices are psychotherapy and pharmacology. Psychotherapy endeavors to have the cerebrum complete handling the awful accident, and utilizing these recollections can revamp the neurotransmitters.

Unlike the compound cracked leg, PTSI doesn't have an unmistakably characterized end-state for treatment. The results of PTSI are abstract to every person. Reliant upon the social-monetary status, culture, and customs, "relieved" shifts essentially from one individual to another. As a rule, there is no last remedy for PTSI, and the singular will have created proper adapting abilities for the executives. All the more significantly, everybody is unique, no two occasions are something similar, and individuals will react contrastingly to various treatments.

The assessed insights for veterans with PTSI change by struggle and by year. The assessed PTSI rates for the Vietnam War are 15%, the Gulf War at 12%, and Iraq/Afghanistan between 11%-20%. As per a RAND Corporation investigation in 2018, roughly 2.8 million assistance individuals have been sent since 9/11/2001. With the above measurements, around

308,000 to 560,000 Iraq and Afghanistan veterans are impacted by PTSI. The pretraumatic factors (sex, schooling, number of arrangements, the part of administration) chances proportion normal is 1.58, while peritraumatic factors (battle openness, releasing weapons, injured and killed) chances proportion normal is
3.03. Indeed, even with an altogether low likelihood of causing PTSI, this injury is outstandingly factor by the person.

umerous elements situated me in Afghanistan of 2006, like family childhood, schooling, mid-west hard working attitudes, and the country's political-societal position. A considerable lot of these characteristics and qualities helped me all through my vocation and organization, and some preparation and convictions permitted endurance without actual injury. By and large, I would survey that the military set me up negligibly for battle. I got the base preparing necessities and expert tutoring. Because of the idea of the public safety technique, the National Guard's entrusting to create and prepare an unfamiliar military was challenging.

The National Guard has a special mission as it plays double parts in the state and the country. Shaped in 1863, it is the longest-serving military in US history. The reason for resident fighters and nearby state armies is to be a prepared power for the Governor and an essential hold power for the country.

The National Guard gave supplemental units into Regular Army units to balance the battle power for every significant conflict. A new model would be the sending of National Guard units for the Desert Storm War. As a local area based association, there was more dependence on the National Guard for prepared powers for the State Governor. Components of the National Guard have been called up into state deployment ready for a considerable length of time, including winter tempests and flooding. Administration in the National Guard can be especially difficult as there are normally under 40 days every year to meet the majority of the preparation necessities as the Regular Army, be ready for state deployment ready, and keep up with non military personnel careers.

I enrolled in 1993, during the essential save time span, preceding President William Clinton instituted, "Don't Ask, Don't Tell." Our unit, alongside numerous other National Guard units, was under-resourced. Our approved strength was low, and we had old gear, missing hardware, and little financing for preparing. Frequently, the National Guard got gear after the Regular Army or accepted their more seasoned things. Preparing during the 90s was one end of the week a month and two weeks per year. The majority of the units directed yearly preparing during the initial fourteen days of June and was

frequently alluded to as day camp as we went through somewhere around ten days in the field at Fort McCoy.

during the 1990s, I didn't anticipate sending to a battle zone. The essential hold implied that we were not relied upon to show up in the battle theater for a very long time after an underlying intrusion. A great deal of preparing and planning would happen after actuation in a future enormous scope war. We had supplemental preparing for state missions by giving security in the jail frameworks in the event of a worker strike. We additionally had revolt control preparing if there should be an occurrence of uproars like the race riots in Milwaukee in the late spring of 1967 when the Governor initiated the National Guard. We focused on our preparation because of the measure of accessible time, ammo, and other restricted assets, and the year's feature was the yearly preparing exercise. Thusly, the attitude was that real battle was a low chance and even lower probability.

Mobilization arranging during the 1990s comprised of fostering an arrangement to move all the work force and gear to the preparation station as a unit. We had numerous folios with phone calling trees, vehicle load cards, preparing plans, and definite designs for food and housing. The essential objective of the exhaustive projects was to guarantee the most measure of staff was prepared, and each and every piece of hardware would get to the battle theater. These plans contained various techniques for taking staff and gear to the battle theater, including airplane, rail, and boat, and how the faculty would connect up with the hardware. I went through hours chipping away at these plans and covers when I was a lesser official. The greater part of my tactical preparing before arrangement moved from field activities to PC based activities. I was expressly prepared in the big guns PC frameworks and invested energy mastering organizing abilities to associate these frameworks. Our ordnance central command advanced its preparation by taking an interest in huge scope PC practices in reproduced fights and wars. Higher central command units facilitated mock fights more than a multi week time spans, and I went to preparing occasions in Germany, South Korea, Fort Lewis, Fort Sheridan, IL, and Fort McCoy. In this way, I had a lot of military preparing facing in reenacted PC conflicts. Programmatic experiences can give preparing to staff capacities and fight following however immensely affect genuine field training.

Shortly after 9/11, the save parts moved from the essential save into a functional power and changed the organization model. After

the Afghanistan and Iraq intrusions, the theater commandants required extra soldiers from the save parts without really wasting any time. A few units and faculty just had a couple of days to tell their boss they were leaving for a year, pack all their tactical attire and some gear, bid farewell to their loved ones and show up at the preparation station. The majority of the short notification activations dismissed the extensive arrangement courses of events and gear preparations.

had an expansive scope of encounters on my sending, particularly as a save field ordnance Captain, and had encounters that many warriors won't have the chance to have. I had tea with Afghan older folks, appreciated Afghan foot bread and rice. I had a translator and taken in a couple of local words and heard the call to petition on the speakers. I had monitor obligation, went on long foot watches, drove firearm trucks, worked automatic weapons on firearm trucks, lived in a weapon truck for quite a long time, flew in Chinook and Blackhawk helicopters, air attacked onto a mountain, been in a base assault, been in a side of the road bomb, and been in various rocket assaults. I cleaned weighty weapons, performed support on the firearm truck, arranged my food, washed my garments, and held up hours to utilize the phone. I had a lot of long stretches of personal time watching motion pictures on my PC and sat in staff gatherings. I smelled the open sewer trenches and consume pits. I additionally shot US big guns, registered the gunnery for Afghan big guns and discharged a short suppressive eruption of an automatic weapon in a firefight on the fifth commemoration of 9/11. I went through hours with the Afghan Army powers getting ready for missions, leading missions, and taking a chance with my life innumerable times.

Training an unfamiliar inner protection is one of the mission sets for the Army Special Forces; nonetheless, with the huge numbers for the staff objective for the Afghanistan Army, customary powers should accept a fundamental job for this mission. In Afghanistan, the tactical order set up a specific team, a gathering of units, with a shared objective of getting sorted out, preparing, and keeping up with the Afghanistan military. In 2003, Regular Army units from the tenth Mountain Division started to lead the pack on building up the team, and inside the year, a National Guard infantry detachment base camp expected the mission. I sent in the fourth turn of faculty. We were entrusted further to extend the Afghanistan Army in the five geographic regions while incorporating it into progressing battle operations.

As a US counsel, I had almost no preparation and altogether less help than the Army Special Forces. A large portion of the consultants were saved component

staff with the second pivot of faculty, enhanced with other supporting countries' tactical powers and different administrations. The vast majority of my preparation before sending was as an essential save power with restricted monitoring and inheritance gear. During our month and a portion of preparation preparing, more often than not was utilized to approve our vital military abilities of weapon acquaintance and capability, clinical screenings, and medical aid. Armed force Special Forces have an exceptionally particular cycle. Preparing requires a very long time to become qualified by finishing exceptionally specific military schools, like Special Forces Qualification Course, language, airborne, air attack, marksman, jumper, and others. Exceptional Forces units got cutting edge hardware and need of help for key resources, while I bought my own Gerber multifunction instrument. I claimed explosives and weapons that I had not prepared on in north of twenty years. I never gotten earlier preparing on certain weapons and frameworks until I utilized them while sent, a learn-as-you-go strategy for training.

A similarity of my arrangement would be somebody finishing a nearby resident's police foundation then, at that point, unexpectedly given the occupation of preparing a FBI moderator during a continuous prisoner emergency talking through a translator. In 2006, our groundwork for mission accomplishment as a battle guide rate was probable in the single digits. We at last had an outlandish mission and had insignificant instruments to deal with achieving what we could. In spite of the chances, I trusted that I could decidedly affect the task.

Rotations and reassignments empowered me to have encounters in a wide cluster of conditions and conditions. I could identify with the fervor levels from the weariness of gatekeeper obligation to being in a firefight. I could allude to severity by living in the field for a week and have restricted conveniences on a base. Be that as it may, others' conflict stories have a repeating theme: the obligation of fellowship and kinship of their colleagues, the shared characteristic of battling for those right close to you and not really for yourself or the mission — the ongoing idea of going to somebody due to the profound trust. I couldn't foster those bonds with anyone.

The climate in the grave eastern locale of Afghanistan was actually and sincerely requesting. The east space of Afghanistan is dry, rocky, dusty, and third-world expectations for everyday comforts. Numerous various families resided in little homes developed with mud and other normal materials. The courses between towns were back roads, ways, and dry riverbeds. Power was scanty, and the web and phone structure barely existed outside of the semi-metropolitan regions. I didn't feel like I could rely upon anybody. For the run of the mill summer battling season months, I was doled out to a little Afghan Army base unit with around two dozen US counsels. While at this base, we had next to no outer help and performed many every day living errands ourselves. The Afghan Army unit gave security at the fundamental door to the base and give security in the lookouts. Our base didn't have any mounted guns, mortars, or radar frameworks. Our base didn't have food administration, vehicle upkeep, or clothing support. The closest US base for outside help was around 15 minutes drive on a back road with potential side of the road bombs. My room on our little base had two different bunkmates who I never settled any association. One bunkmate was an individual Captain, Weist, and the other bunkmate was a lesser official. These officials had staff occupations for faculty and coordinations the executives and were not entrusted to go on numerous missions or watches because of the absence of confidence in their capacities. Consequently, our timetable didn't synchronize, and I didn't invest a lot of energy with either one.

On the one hand, it was great to be away from the obsessively hovering over base camp, yet then again, this far off task made a semi-defenseless inclination as we depended on others for any help. We would need to drive 15 minutes to the US base to get food and some vehicle parts, and afterward we cooked for us and kept up with our vehicles. Notwithstanding the self-life support capacities, we gave administration and mentorship to the Afghan Army troopers by leading practically every day battle watches and missions.

Being in so many exact approaching rocket assaults felt massively vulnerable. After the approaching rockets progressed from disturbance to risk, I felt serious sensations of escaping or submitting. The main thing you can do upon the underlying rocket assault is to caution others and quickly look for cover. In a rocket assault, utilizing your gun or rifle is completely ineffectual. You are dependent that some different powers can draw in the rocket dispatch point, generally with US big guns shoot. I was so restless to leave one base as I had numerous contemplations that one of the rockets would have grievous occasions for me as it was inevitable. Many battle veterans would prefer to be in a firefight gone against to a rocket or mortar assault as there is a chance to react. As a US consultant, I regularly depended on others for help and protection.

Nighttime in Afghanistan is incredibly dull. Outside of Kabul, I didn't see any streetlamps, and numerous Afghan homes were lit with candles or oil lights because of the absence of power. Curfews would forestall vehicles from

going around evening time with headlights. All bases kept up with power outage conditions, implying that individuals couldn't utilize white electric lamps or headlights. Every one of the windows were covered to limit light outflow from the room. A base in power outage conditions creates a troublesome objective for the foe and disguises the base's movement. An individual could utilize a little, pen-sized red or green light to stroll around the base as these lights are hard to see from a brief distance. Despite the fact that rooms had lights and I could utilize red or green lights, it was as yet important to have a little white spotlight for flagging, see something rapidly in the truck, or other fast employments. I generally had a shaded light cut to my uniform top and a little white spotlight in my uniform top pocket. I likewise had additional shaded lights for my shorts to get to the washroom at night.

Tracers help the shooter's point in discharging rifles and automatic weapons around evening time. Be that as it may, tracer adjusts go the two different ways, as it will likewise distinguish the shooter's situation to the adversary. There is no standard with tracer adjusts in that all adversary tracers are red, and cordial tracers are green. There are different shades of tracer adjusts, to incorporate infrared tracers noticeable just with night vision gadgets. When seeing any tracers with night vision goggles, it shows up as a rapidly moving radiant green speck. It tends to trick to witness a firefight around evening time with tracers as it appears to be that the shooting is slow; notwithstanding, truly, there are four projectiles between each tracer round that you can't see, and tracers have restricted distances of brightening.

y most recent couple of months was throughout the colder time of year and was filled generally with outrageous weariness. I was in Gardez and I was excited to move away from Bermel with the rocket assaults. My last occupation was not a set up position, so I wound up chipping away at odd tasks. My different undertakings didn't need a lot of time, so I had a long time of with lots but idle time. Maybe the schedule paused and time hauled out. Going to the fair suppers was a feature of the day.

Three quarters into my organization, I was restless to return home and didn't have any desire to be there any longer. It was cold outside, and there was nothing to do other than lounge around your bunk region. I experienced difficulty resting around evening time, and I heard that a lesser fighter saw a battle pressure individual a couple of months earlier and had gotten a solution for dozing. Another US consultant recommended going to the on-base clinical treatment community to get Benadryl for a tranquilizer. At the point when I showed up at the treatment place and informed them what I needed, they finished an underlying appraisal, and the Physician Assistant conversed with me. I left the treatment community with a stock of Benadryl and a duplicate of

my admission evaluation structure, which I immediately annihilated as I didn't need anybody to be aware of my rest issue. A long time later, while going through the retirement interaction, I shockingly saw a duplicate of this screening structure in my tactical clinical records.

Beginning the redeployment cycle is invigorating as it is nearly an ideal opportunity to return home. As redeployment is a tactical interaction, there are many advances, sub-cycles, and postponements. With the energy development, there is likewise a high craving to traverse the cycle as fast as could really be expected. With the craving to overcome quickly, there is solid protection from unveil whatever could create extra setbacks. Assuming somebody uncovers a physical issue that happened during arrangement, there is a decent possibility that you would need to remain behind to get assessed and treated.

At the deactivation station upon get back from Afghanistan, I went through a few stations to out-process. One of the stations was for starting cases with the Department of Veterans Affairs for inability. Since I was in a functioning status, I could just have the delegate check the square that I was available at their table as the tactical medical coverage would cover any necessary consideration. Clinical screening was most of the out-handling focus. A portion of the clinical stations were normal screenings, like tuberculous and hearing. I finished an internet based survey, the post-arrangement wellbeing evaluation that contained conventional inquiries of openness to the climate (residue, radiation, and smoke) and nonexclusive inquiries concerning openness to battle (seeing dead bodies and discharge weapons). I met with a clinical specialist to audit every one of the outcomes and the post-organization wellbeing evaluation. I was exceptionally specific on things I uncovered as I needed to get back as booked and try not to turn into a remnant. I showed that I saw dead bodies and shot my weapon, however rejected further assessment to keep the cycle moving.

I had at first idea that the side of the road bomb assault was my horrendous mishap. By God's beauty, I was truly unharmed, despite the fact that I was an uncovered heavy armament specialist in the truck, and the blast encompassed us. I possibly saw dark and dim when I looked behind me. In the wake of turning the truck around, and getting back to the site, I saw waiting dark smoke, smelled the mix of the blast, tissue, and residue, and saw a body lying close to a hole in the country road. I additionally dreaded to do medical aid as it had been some time since preparing and figured it would be simpler to utilize the reason of remaining on my automatic rifle to assist with security. I could recognize my reaction to act, as I didn't run

away, and I didn't participate in the reaction. I didn't have overpowering feelings over the passings in the side of the road bomb assault, yet I felt like I ought to have accomplished more than assisting with security. As our truck was nearest to the blast site, I was very quickly the edge's deepest part. There was no requirement for our weapon truck to have a monitored assault rifle as the Afghan warriors immediately went to the strategic position around us.

ver time, I understood my staggering feelings and reactions are identified with the night base assault rather than the side of the road bomb assault. I had more grounded sensations of being ill-equipped and deserted. The side of the road bomb assault likely left a PTSI engrave, particularly with the sentiments that I ought to have accomplished more. I accept that remaining in the truck was the best spot to stow away and keep away from some other risks or getting my hands canvassed in blood. During the base assault, I reacted to the "approaching" yells by rapidly putting on my body protective layer and cap and getting to the fortification. I was neglectful of what was going on around me. At the point when I left the safe house, I felt so alone and deserted. My brain went clear on any activities, and I felt detached. I was unable to track down anybody, and when I tracked down somebody, nobody appeared to notice or take responsibility of me. No one minded that I was going around without help from anyone else without my weapon in my shorts and shirt. I could distinguish my actual reaction to submit, as I was ill-equipped, and I depended on others instructing me. Intellectually, I was in flight mode as I needed just to getaway.

Words can't communicate the feelings I had that evening. It was an exceptional deserting, seclusion, deficiency, ineptness, nonsensical, and not esteemed. The most clear scene that evening was the point at which I went to the Afghan Army side of the base. I had on my boots, shorts, shirt, body reinforcement, gun, cap, and night vision goggles. I had left the fortification, understanding that no other person went to the haven. I had recently run past the billeting rooms, and I saw no other US counselors. I just passed through the little entryway into the Afghan Army compound. I was utilizing my night vision goggles, so everything was a mix of grainy greens and blacks. I could see green tracer shots shooting in various ways overhead. I could see extraordinary, dazzling green glimmers and hear momentary blasts and machine gunfire. I saw a couple of Afghan Army warriors going around and getting more ammo boxes from their capacity holders. I frantically didn't have any desire to be there. I immediately understood that I was unable to address the Afghan Army officers as I was without my mediator, so I kept silent. My psyche went clear with alarm and could

not consider what to do or where to go. I have never felt so disengaged and deserted. After the other US consultant recommended we go to the activities community, I felt unreasonable. I never considered going to the activities community. The essential Army fight drills and good judgment got away my mind.

THE GOOD

"Don't allow your battle to turn into your personality." –

The two main medical treatment programs for PTSI are psychotherapy and pharmacology. PTSI and treatment options are individualistic and may require one or both medical treatments or other alternatives. Different ways of dealing with stress will effectsly affect individuals. I consider reasonable methods for dealing with stress to lessen the uneasiness or misery manifestations and deal with the general effect of this injury. Everybody will have their singular administration techniques.

PSYCHOTHERAPY

Cognitive-conduct treatment and delayed openness treatment are by and large suggested as first-line medicines for PTSI and have a viability pace of 60%. The three primary objectives of treatment are to further develop indications, foster adapting abilities, reestablish confidence, and be individual meetings or in a social environment. The essential treatment is intellectual handling treatment, where you talk about the horrible accident and learn better approaches to reside with it. Delayed openness and eye development desensitization and reprocessing treatments are additionally valuable. Commonly, I am a consistent scholar, and conduct wellbeing has been a secret region for me to comprehend. I lived outside of the separation from the tactical clinics. I was in dynamic military status, so I utilized the tactical medical coverage to get therapy with my regular citizen specialist. On my next regular checkup in mid 2017, I illuminated my clinical specialist about my conversation with the advisor, and she alluded me to conduct health.

At my first treatment arrangement, I was really restless. I never had a treatment arrangement, so I didn't have the foggiest idea what's in store, how to talk,

what the specialist records in notes, and who might be familiar with my issue. I discovered that my advisor was additionally a conduct wellbeing expert with the National Guard. Her tactical experience was advantageous to me as she knew about the association, construction, missions, and wording. Furthermore, she knew about battle PTSI, where regular citizen conduct wellbeing staff may just interface with PTSI from sexual injury or mishaps. Regularly, regular citizens get mistaken and lost for military wording, and I want to clarify things. After my fifth meeting, my specialist informed me that she was passing on to seek after another vocation opportunity. We examined proceeding with treatment with another specialist, yet I was reluctant with regards to continuing with treatment meetings. I felt that I had a superior comprehension of what I was going through, and I needed to keep my uneasiness and PTSI issues to myself.

At the start of 2018, I conversed with my clinical specialist concerning how I was all the while battling, and she alluded me to conduct wellbeing once more. I was getting help meetings for about a year. A considerable lot of the treatment meetings were intellectual handling based, and I had five meetings for eye development desensitization and reprocessing treatment. During these treatment meetings, I additionally had composed openness treatment, which was the basis for First to Fire. My subsequent specialist had no tactical experience; notwithstanding, I felt like I was advancing through treatment as she was completely qualified and authorized to treat the source problem.

There are benefits and burdens to having an advisor with military experience. The particular benefit is that they know the phrasing and culture. As a patient, I didn't feel like I expected to make an interpretation of the military talk into regular citizen talk. The vast majority of the regular citizen populace has no openness to military life and culture, so I feel like I really want to change over the tactical phrasing into more clear terms. Rather than saying, "I was on a GAC in our UAH to the FOB, and we hit an IED," I would want to convert into saying, "I was on a caravan in our defensively covered weapon truck to the base, and we hit a side of the road bomb." However, I some way or another felt that my advisor with military experience was passing judgment on me. I realize that she was not making a decision about me, however it made me uncomfortable as I was an Army official in treatment for encounters that happened years prior, and some way or another, I ought to be over this problem.

My specialist suggested attempting eye development desensitization and reprocessing. I have never known about this sort of treatment. She clarified that I

would advance through two or three phases by first recognizing a protected spot and afterward talking through the horrendous mishap while watching her fingers go this way and that. My first task was to distinguish a protected spot that I could allude back to during future medicines, like perusing a book on the ocean front on a radiant day. The protected spot ought to be where it makes you cheerful and loose. While the ocean side scene is great, I don't want to be out in the immediate sun as I burn from the sun without any problem. I experienced difficulty thinking about my protected spot. I reviewed an exceptionally quiet scene when I was a lesser ordnance official. I had recently finished the computations and coordination for a perplexing enlightenment mission, and I sat on top of our followed vehicle in the murkiness, watching the howitzers terminating. Everything was going without a hitch, and I had an enthusiastic high from the feeling of achievement. In any case, dim and blasts would not be a suggested safe spot during PTSI directing. I chose being at my little girl's swim meet as it was inside, warm, the smell of the pool, and pleased with watching my girl swimming admirably. At the following guiding meeting, I utilized the swimming scene, however it caused some nervousness and fervor as it was a competition.

My advisor and I endeavored to change the scene somewhat by envisioning my girl simply completing the occasion in any case, and afterward there was consistently the following race. I chose to change sees for my protected spot. My protected spot scene is me cutting my grass on a shady day. I partake in the spotless lines and progress. I appreciate paying attention to music on my earphones with the steady foundation commotion from the lawnmower motor. My main cooperation with individuals as they drove by is a straightforward wave. I partake in the smell of new cut grass and wouldn't fret the work and getting somewhat filthy. The eye development desensitization and reprocessing treatment itself burrows profound and attempts to outline the feelings felt during the occasion and even review portions of the occasion that possibly the psyche has hindered. It was about this time when I began expounding on my horrible mishap. After the second or third meeting, I felt like I mistakenly depicted something during the gathering, so I composed notes about it. In the following meeting, my specialist had me perused my notes out loud.

I proceeded with a portion of my schoolwork tasks after treatment. I keep on making child strides for social circumstances, which assist with breaking the detachment obstruction. I pushed my usual range of familiarity to work on my confidence as a journalist for a Milwaukee TV channel reached me through Facebook Messenger asking assuming I would have a meeting with him. Now, I had just expounded on my horrible encounters, and just verbally talked

about them with my specialist. This news report was extremely effective for me as I had tension with regards to the meeting viewpoints and expressing my occasions before the general public.

any veterans track down some solace in talking among different veterans as a type of treatment. There are imparted convictions and culture to veterans, and they can without much of a stretch identify with battle encounters. Chatting with different veterans who had a similar encounter and in similar fights and guards can for sure be advantageous. For my situation, while I was composing First to Fire, it was exclusively from my notes, pictures, and memory. I momentarily met up with two or three others in similar commitment on my sending and got their point of view on the occasion, which filled in certain openings in what I couldn't remember.

PHARMACOLOGY

Some patients either don't react enough or favor drugs. Specific serotonin reuptake inhibitors sorts of antidepressants have a reaction pace of roughly 60%, with better outcomes with the blend of psychotherapy. The objective of pharmacology is to adjust the synapses inside the mind. Drugs can assist with having an uplifting perspective on life and assist with feeling typical. Sertraline, a specific serotonin reuptake inhibitor, is commonly recommended as a first preliminary to start pharmacology. Sertraline has not many aftereffects and is thought of as powerful. Sertraline is a stimulant, and the Food and Drug Administration endorsed the medicine for PTSI treatment. Sertraline is intended to change the serotonin levels inside the cerebrum. It doesn't deliver a high inclination, however it brings some relief as I don't feel the outrageous tension sentiments. As far as I might be concerned, sertraline removed the elevated sea tide and diminished the meaning of the waves.

There are different antidepressants accessible, and relying upon what other ailments an individual has may likewise influence the sort and dose of the medication. I remained on a similar drug, and I adjusted the measurement a couple of times. I was available to drug therapy dependent on the suggestion from my clinical specialist. I have been on every day medicine for elevated cholesterol for a really long time, so it would not be very different assuming that I really wanted a solution to adjust my cerebrum's science. I asked my primary care physician how long I would be on sertraline, and her reaction was estimated in years.

UNNING

Running can further develop an individual's actual wellness levels and can deliver positive endorphins. I tracked down racing to unwinding and pleasant. It was forty

minutes of decompression and a psychological reset. Very quickly after redeployment in 2007, I began running. I saw a companion running, and I felt that I should run more to be cutthroat with him. The Army actual wellness test comprised of two minutes of push-ups, two minutes of sit-ups, and a two-mile run. I have consistently scored between the base and most extreme scores however imagined that running would improve me position me for my next task. It was a hard beginning, starting with two miles multi week and gradually adding one more day and minimal longer distances. Throughout the colder time of year, I ran on the treadmills in the cellar, watching the nearby news. When I begin working in Madison in the fall of 2009, I was running five miles each work day and up to ten miles on Fridays. Running turned into my thing. I had bought fair running shoes and had exceptional shorts, jeans, shirts, and coats. At the point when I began running, I paid attention to music on my computerized media player yet before long tracked down that diverting. I delighted in running, being outside, and seeing the sights, and paying attention to the sounds around me, particularly down the Oak Leaf Trail way in Milwaukee and the Starkweather Creek way in Madison.

In 2010, I felt exceptionally certain and happy with running. Despite the fact that I have not run in excess of ten miles, I was certain I could run a long distance race. I pursued my very first running race, the 2010 Madison Marathon on Memorial Day weekend. With time imperatives, I couldn't finish a preparation run for longer than 14 miles. Notwithstanding, during that 14-mile preparing run, I had the option to keep an eight-minute mile pace. My essential objective in the long distance race was to finished the occasion, with an auxiliary objective of time under four hours and a tertiary objective of running the whole course. Tragically, the climate on Memorial Day weekend set record highs, and the race authorities dark hailed the occasion because of temperatures in the upper 90s. Despite the fact that the race authorities urged members to board transports at the water stations, I needed to finish it. I had the option to remain with my unique running gathering for the initial 18 miles before I began strolling breaks. A few homes towards the finish of the race set up sprinklers in the street and utilized hoses to splash the sprinters. With my throbbing feet and the weariness from the hotness, I immediately changed to strolling more than running. I completed the Madison Marathon in 4 hours and 22 minutes, accomplishing my essential objective however missed the mark regarding my auxiliary goals.

RITING

Written account openness treatment helped me the most. As a

contemplative person and utilizing withdrawal for adapting, I observed the most ideal method for putting myself out there was composing. I could take as much time as necessary and be more genuine and open, without the dread of quick judgment that you can get with verbal correspondence. I could compose notes at work during my lunch or compose on my iPad while my little girl was at swim practice. Composing is a tranquil and smart cycle. Writing in an electronic archive likewise permits changes and can rapidly begin and stop. Composing can be extremely close to home, and the author can pick what to share and what not to share and with whom to share.

After I distributed First to Fire, my significant other inquired as to whether I expounded on everything from my sending. I didn't depict each film I watched for sure I ate at every dinner, except there were stories that I at first composed and eliminated during the altering system. Some portion of the creative cycle is to know your crowd, henceforth the insignificant utilization of military vernacular inside this distribution. You can have a composing style for yourself, such as keeping a journal, a composing style for correspondence with companions or family, similar to email correspondence, or a composing style for a more extensive crowd. Between treatment meetings, I expounded on my awful accidents a few times, adding more subtleties and portraying the tangible climate. After I generally finished tales about my awful mishaps, I kept on composition as it was a method for articulating my thoughts purposely, and I expounded on other critical occasions during my arrangement. I kept on adding to my brief tales by adding foundation data and what life resembled in that somber region in 2006. The vast majority of my works now were for my memory and to impart to my therapist.

As I kept on composition, I understood that this would be a magnificent medium to unite my dispersing of documented data. I had many computerized pictures put away on one hard drive, chronicled messages put away in a reinforcement document, an every day schedule with bulleted features saved in a record that would turn out of date, and I had recollections put away in my mind that would gradually disappear. I understood that I could keep on expounding on my arrangement, and I would have the option to assemble the entire story with this large number of wellsprings of data to foster a solitary source. I likewise needed to have the option to impart my organization story to my girl and family. My little girl was 11 years of age at that point, so I needed her to have the story when she was age-suitable. I composed my story in a record. I added various pictures; be that as it may, the size of the archive was extensive and would be hard to share, so I investigated diverse printing choices and chose to independently publish a book through

Amazon. Amazon has an extraordinary program that permits self-distribution of books with soft cover and Kindle forms and permits me to impart my story to loved ones without any problem. I took in an extraordinary arrangement about composition, altering, sentence structure, and formatting.

MAN'S BEST FRIEND

My significant other and I have not been pet individuals while we have been hitched, and our little girl just had a goldfish for Christmas one year. After tirelessness from our little girl, we at last broke to get a doggy. Our girl went through hours exploring and looking at changed varieties, and her top suggestion was a Maltipoo, a blend of Maltese and toy poodle. Her benefits for a Maltipoo were hypoallergenic, little, great with youngsters, and effectively teachable. At the point when we chose to purchase a Maltipoo from a raiser, we were unable to find a reproducer in Wisconsin. We tracked down a reproducer in Toledo, Ohio, and we put down a little store to get on the holding up list. Timing on getting the little dog would be a colossal deterrent as the raiser didn't have a clue when our name would come up on the shortlist and the number of pups showed up in each litter. Also, Toledo is around ten hours of heading out and had school and work schedules.

Meanwhile, we saw that our neighbor had new little dogs and found that she accepted her pups from a reproducer close to Saint Louis, Missouri. We looked into that reproducer on the web and saw that she had a very adorable cream-hued Maltipoo that would be accessible in half a month and would be under nine pounds when completely developed. We immediately dedicated and saw that a couple from West Bend, Wisconsin was taking on one more Maltipoo in the litter. A few was anticipating heading to Saint Louis for pickup. We facilitated with the West Bend couple to have our doggy shipped home, saving us long periods of driving. We immediately expected to sort out the best supplies to buy and as soon as possible get familiar with the rudiments of really focusing on a puppy.

Having another pup in the house subsequent to being non-pet individuals was without a doubt loaded with difficulties. At the point when we initially got Molly, she brought consideration that another little dog brings among the neighbors and passers-by. While she was pup preparing and getting to get familiar with our home, I invested energy outside as it was exceptionally great out in right on time to mid-June. Nearly everybody that drove, trekked, or strolled by our home halted to see the new little dog. Being outside without help from anyone else was not my inclination as I would prefer to be in the house to stay away from individuals, yet constrained me to have wonderful good tidings with the neighbors and meet some new individuals. I would require in excess of a wave to somebody passing by, as they would ask my doggy's name, breed, and age, which constrained me into little talk.

Molly benefited and console me the most, and she is the ideal pet for our family. I have concentrated on her as she is reliant upon me for taking care of, strolling, and playing. She gets so eager to see me when I return home, and she cuddles facing me around evening time before bed. Unqualified love. Despite the fact that she at times makes hardships with planning, I anticipate returning home and going for her for a stroll or playing. I would frequently sit outside in the front yard with Molly on pleasant days for quite a long time at a time, as she particularly loves to pursue blowing leaves. I would go for Molly on long strolls through our area, which assisted with speaking with different neighbors. At the point when I began our strolls, I immediately scholarly of practically every one of the canine's names in the area, and I began talking more to their proprietors. Molly is generally honored by an amazing neighbor who really focuses on her while we work during the day. My better half and I are appreciative to have Molly impart her satisfaction and love to a sort and liberal neighbor.

have not looked for true assignment of Molly as a passionate help creature. In Wisconsin, a passionate help creature can be practically any creature; as a rule, canines and felines that can furnish solace to people with despondency, tension, and PTSI, and requires a solution from a psychological well-being proficient. While Molly offers me incredible solace and loves to be with her all the more regularly, an assignment of passionate help creatures, just permits assurances with lodging and air travel. Enthusiastic help creatures might help people that lease or have successive air travel; but since Molly as of now resides in my home, and I scarcely fly, there isn't a craving to look for true assignment. Passionate help creatures are not managed the cost of a similar scope as assigned assistance creatures in open buildings.

FAITH AND RELIGION

When I was youthful, I tried different things with a few unique religions and houses of worship. I went to a few Confraternity of Christian Doctrine classes, going to a Baptist church, and wound up with the Evangelical Lutheran Church in America and affirmed as Lutheran. I was acknowledged and go to Marquette University, which is a Jesuit Catholic college. I had an altercation with my congregation and had no cooperation in chapel gatherings and battled with religious philosophy classes. I met my future spouse during my freshman year, and during my school years, I went to Catholic Mass with her a couple of times. During our commitment, I went through the Rite of Christian Initiation of Adults for the Catholic Church. We had a customary Catholic wedding; notwithstanding, our participation at Mass subsequently was inconsistent. My better half gave me a Saint Christopher emblem before organization, and I kept it from that point onward with my tactical distinguishing proof tags.

I went to a short Mass in Manas Air Force Base in Kyrgyzstan while going to Afghanistan and a Mass in French in Kabul, Afghanistan, upon appearance. I generally kept the plastic Rosary that I got in the Kabul house of prayer after the Mass in French in my shoulder pocket of my fight uniform. I attempted to discuss the Hail Mary supplication before I nodded off around evening time. While sent, I didn't approach a Chaplain until the most recent few months in Gardez. There was one Catholic Chaplain in our space, and he went to our base for Mass assistance once every a long time, yet the beginning occasions vacillated because of the accessibility of transportation. He held Mass in an unfilled B-Hut with plastic seats and a collapsing table for an Alter. Around six to twelve people joined in, and we read everything without singing, including the Responsorial Psalms. The Chaplain ordinarily came on Sundays, yet Sundays were normally standard working days. Our regular down day was Friday, as this was the Muslim comparable to Sunday. It was great to get the Host and Blood and to have this individual reflection time.

While my better half and I lived in Watertown, we went to Mass a couple of times yet never settled a decent association with that congregation. At the point when we moved to Oconomowoc, we joined Saint Jerome Parish and had a profound association. The congregation building was worked in 2008 and was lovely and had a significant plan. It is a really noteworthy structure with an appended school that our girl would have the option to go to through eighth grade. Both of our clerics have been exceptionally steady of the military and veterans. Our first minister customarily gave the Invocation at the City of Oconomowoc's metro recognition every Memorial Day. He said this occasion was tied for first as his features during the year. At Mass every week, he likewise gave an extraordinary gift for military help individuals. He adjusted the petition said over individuals during Our Mother of Perpetual Help dedications. Toward the finish of the supplication for expectations, all parishioners would lift their hands in gift the military. He would present, "May the Lord Jesus Christ be with them, that He might shield them, inside them that He might support them, before them that He might lead them, behind them that He might ensure them, above them that He

might favor them for the sake of the Father, the Son, and the Holy Spirit. Amen."

Our new cleric has a unique association with the military as he helped at the United States Naval Academy before in his ministry. While he was the minister in Eagle River, AK, a significant number of his parishioners were military faculty and families from neighboring Joint Base Elmendorf-Richardson. I was acknowledged into the Catholic Church just about twenty years prior, and my confidence is imperative to me. I attempt to carry on with my life morally and ethically as indicated by my beliefs.

INVOLVEMENT

One of my schoolwork tasks from treatment was to have casual conversation with another person. I struggled moving toward this on the grounds that, during standard swim rehearses, I would place in my earphones and pay attention to a book recording or watch a show on my iPad. I saw one more parent that normally remained in the cheap seats during swim practice. Following a long time, I at last took out my earphones and did the off-kilter presentation, and we had a casual conversation for some time. I discovered that her youngsters would go to my girl's school to have extra commonality.

As my girl is getting more established, she is turning out to be more into sports. I had felt that our uncommon bond was gone, however it has quite recently changed. I assist with schoolwork, particularly math and science, and I was associated with scoring for every one of her games. I may not have the foggiest idea about the game all around ok to mentor or to be a line-type judge, however I appreciate keeping up with the authority records. I'm an affirmed USA Swimming Administrative Official dependable to the Referee and responsible for the exact handling of sections, scratches, and cultivating and deciding and recording official occasions. I'm the substitute scorekeeper for our select softball and am a scorekeeper for grade school ball and volleyball. There are a lot of freedoms to reach out, wilt in sports, school, veterans' gatherings, metro networks, holy places, and a large group of different associations and events.

REINTEGRATION AND RESILIENCY

Over the most recent ten years, the military took jumps and limits stressing reintegration from sending and showing fighters flexibility abilities. Our state National Guard base camp set up a reintegration program in

September 2006. The purpose is to rapidly build up the returning veteran and their close family with assets that might help him/her with their progress. The primary gathering was held a few months after redeployment

and incorporated a family reintegration instructions. Each help part and their relatives met secretly with delegates from every one of the accompanying associations: Chaplain, maintenance, Military and Family Life Consultant, Vet Centers, Employer Support of the Guard and Reserve, legitimate, State Veterans Benefits Advisor, County Veteran Service Office, Inspector General, State Youth Coordinator, and the Wisconsin State Family Program Coordinator. Our organization bunch from Wisconsin had a Yellow Ribbon invite service at the Chula Vista Resort in Wisconsin Dells. It was one of the initial gatherings to process through the program. Every one of us was permitted to bring a huge other for a private service on a Friday night, staying short-term, and go through the majority of the day on Saturday going through reintegration preparing with our better half. There was no an ideal opportunity to partake in the waterpark at the hotel, however the retreat gave huge house type rooms at the contracted rate. The service was short, and the state initiative gave each a banner, coin, and a couple of different knickknacks. The 2008 National Defense Authorization Act set up the authority Yellow Ribbon Reintegration Program and became Public Law 110-181. The program gives occasions that interface troopers and their families with neighborhood data on medical services, schooling openings, and monetary and legitimate benefits.

Around 2010, the Army carried out the flexibility program. As the official responsible for our unit, I expected to distinguish an officer to go to dominate strength preparing at the University of Pennsylvania. I didn't have a clue what strength was, and I chose an officer who had great actual wellness test scores and had the option to go to the course for quite some time. Upon her return, I discovered that the program was tied in with building fundamental abilities. The Army in the long run began having compulsory preparing quarterly to learn flexibility. Warriors in fundamental preparing get flexibility preparing, and boost preparing happens over time to support these transient abilities. The versatility program is like positive reasoning treatment or intellectual conduct treatment to supplant negative considerations with positive musings. There are 14 absolute modules for the total versatility program that the University of Pennsylvania created: Activating Event and Consequences module helps fabricate mindfulness. Chase the Good Stuff module helps construct idealism and positive feelings, and Mental Games changes the concentrate away from counterproductive thinking.

GUIDED MEDITATION

My first advisor proposed that I attempt reflection to help unwind, suggest a web-based contemplation program, and gave several different strategies for unwinding. I comprehend the idea of reflection and the advantages of clearing your brain, profound breathing, and unwinding; nonetheless, I was unable to remain on track. My psyche meandered, and I was stressed over counting for the appropriate period of time. There are positively medical advantages to reflection and yoga and may even be sufficient to diminish nervousness levels. Contemplation might be a helpful positive method for dealing with stress to diminish uneasiness symptoms.

MINDFULNESS

One of the most recent PTSI the executives abilities is care. Care includes thoughtful and mind-body rehearses and advances unwinding and serenity and has been in presence for a really long time in the old East. Care lessens nervousness and assists individuals with zeroing in on the present. The objective of care is to awaken to the internal activities of our psychological, enthusiastic, and actual cycles. Applying care to PTSI is a generally more up to date approach and is under research. Care goes past reflection and joins the body. Compelling care requires the act of a few abilities. Mindfulness is concentrating on each thing in turn and perceiving everything around you. Nonjudgmental perception eliminates the great and awful names of encounters. Being right now is being a functioning member instead of making an insincere effort. At long last, the fledgling's psyche is opening up to new encounters and changes.

BREATHING

One of the most regular and most economical methods for dealing with stress are straightforward breathing activities. Lieutenant Colonel Dave Grossman, a conspicuous previous Special Forces fighter who showed brain research at West Point, is a tremendous promoter for showing this breathing activity for officials in the field. He's prepared military pilots and decidedly affects their feelings of anxiety during rapid pursuits. At the point when you're in an endurance attitude, it's difficult to consider whatever else. However, research shows that battle breathing is a viable method for dealing with the adrenaline dump of energy and nerves from the pressure.

he equation for battle breathing is straightforward: Breathe in through your nose for a count of four, pause your breathing for a count of four, breathe out through your mouth for a count of four, and pause your breathing again for a count of four. Restart the cycle however many occasions as fundamental. It's fundamental for attempt to fill and

void your lungs with every period. Inhale profoundly and permit your psyche to zero in on the breath. Permit the nerves to stream out with the breathe out and permit your body to balance out notwithstanding the adrenaline rush.

Combat breathing, as other breath control procedures, is a way for you to reset your sensory system and carefully check in with your body. It breaks the snapshot of pressure and permits you to flood your body with the oxygen it needs as it kicks into acute stress mode.

It's additionally one of the quicker breathing procedures as far as availability. All you really want is your breath, and the recipe is easy to recollect. In an increased mental state — regardless of whether Special Forces or regular citizen — it's useful to have an apparatus that will assist you with tracking down your direction back to quiet. Research has shown that dialing back your breath battles the pressure reaction and can diminish your pulse and blood pressure.

THE BAD

"All of us are broken somehow, some hold the pieces together better." – Anonymous

The list of bad or harmful coping strategies is long. Many of these mechanisms can quickly degrade and develop into additional anxiety or depression or continue into severe addictions.

WITHDRAWAL AND ISOLATION

Withdrawal is the negative method for dealing with stress that impacted me the most, and it required a long time to perceive. I promptly said the inclination was to be separated from everyone else as I was a contemplative person. Lamentably, a large number of my aversion practices probably prompted my vocation level. I unequivocally liked to work autonomously and endeavored to keep away from gatherings and gathering projects. I didn't draw in myself with the social parts of work, for example, interpersonal interaction, and functions. I applied for a couple of advancement openings, for the most part since I thought I expected to advance in my vocation; in any case, I kept away from extra obligations and better standards. With my powerful urge to stay secluded, the view of me was that I was not putting forth a concentrated effort, and I was not prepared for places of expanded responsibility.

I went after a few jobs in the following higher grade when I was qualified. There were places that I was capable for, and numerous associates imagined that I would be a programmed choice. For every one of the six positions that I applied for, I contemplated, ready, and thought about my traits. The choosing bosses said I progressed nicely, yet another person was better and typically some remark about being more sure or planning more. Unnoticed at that point, I had serious uneasiness about these meetings, with a dread of judgment, dismissal, and insufficiencies. I review one meeting that the first

question was "inform us concerning yourself." I felt my heart beating, face becoming red, I got limited focus, and I can't recollect what I muttered for a reply.

I'm a contemplative person and favor a couple of companions. Be that as it may, throughout the long term, I had no genuine companions past my better half. I have numerous associates and expert connections, however I didn't have anybody I could go to in a period of scarcity. Nobody has any complaints against me, and I share an agreeable grin and perhaps a "hi." There is few associates whom I feel happy with having casual conversation. Different guardians from my girl's school, guardians, mentors from sports, and neighbors are all acquaintances.

sooner or later in 2017, somebody remarked that I may have social uneasiness. In the wake of surveying the condition, I felt like I met the majority of the manifestations, particularly: low confidence, low feeling of privilege, execution nervousness; self-judgment; ridiculous assumptions toward yourself; and individuals pleasing

– an inordinate requirement for acknowledgment or endorsement among others. In any event, during a short conversation with my significant other, she said that she might have let me know that I had social nervousness. I conversed with my non military personnel clinical specialist again about the chance of social nervousness and a portion of my manifestations. She alluded me back to directing. After my underlying evaluation, my primary care physician prescribed and endorsed prescription to decrease nervousness manifestations. After a couple of directing meetings, I understood that I didn't have social nervousness however was utilizing withdrawal as an adapting mechanism.

all things being equal, my awareness of others' expectations diminished altogether since my powerlessness to act fittingly the evening of the base assault. I stayed away from obligation at the side of the road bomb assault and different activities on sending. I thought I put in a critical energy in arranging and leading the activity's calculated perspectives. I assumed the job of a manager two or three years after arrangement, however I regarded that occupation as a placeholder, and I zeroed in on running. I did well in positions in a help job and ceaselessly excelled on my assessments, yet I tried not to look for occupations with prominent places and assumptions. It is hard to advance in the military assuming you stay away from responsibility.

COMPARTMENTALIZATION

Compartmentalization is regularly considered to be a negative component as it is the subliminal mental guard to stay away from intellectual discord or nervousness. The capacity for the psyche to close on one occasion and move onto the following can be an incredible resource during battle. The mission necessities frequently don't allow

time to harp on occasions. For example, your fight mate turns into a loss while an infantry group is assaulting a dugout, there is no an ideal opportunity to harp on how their life will be changed, how their family will be impacted, nor think about the happy occasions together ahead of time. Your fight pal needs medical aid, and the group actually needs to assault the dugout. Compartmentalization permits the trooper to proceed with the mission. While compartmentalization is useful for the battle trooper, it influences psychological wellness and makes me lose some passionate associations with individuals. I don't for the most part ponder my sending, and there are numerous parts of my organization that I have not contemplated since it happened.

If living could be introduced on a course of events from - 5 (living previously) to 0 (embracing the here and now) to +5 (living later on), I would quite often be a

4, with a periodic - 3 negative musings and recollections. I have an intrinsic need to know what's next. I keep a definite schedule and get disappointed assuming something comes up unscheduled. I plan menus for the week and simply go to the supermarket one time each week, and I am continually asking my better half what I should make for supper the following little while. On our last family get-away to Walt Disney World in Florida, I had transportation, dinners, and Fast Passes generally planned to the moment to amplify our time there. While partaking in the Seven Dwarfs Mine Train rollercoaster, I was pondering getting to the following ride.

Compartmentalization had a negative part of my associations with loved ones. Probably my dearest companion and flat mates in school was the best person for my wedding. We got together a few times a short time later, yet life disrupted everything. Nothing adverse occurred between us. I continued on, and unfortunately, I have not pondered him for quite a long time. Compartmentalization made a figurative agenda for my life as I generally have things on my rundown, get confirmed, and afterward continued on to the following thing. I was ceaselessly assessed profoundly for specialized information and having an incredible memory. I effectively review what Army guideline applies to what in particular process and can review subjects talked about in a tactical school from quite a while prior. I would have the option to set up a gunnery outline today, which I have not done in very nearly 20 years, however I can't remember any names of companions from essential preparing or fundamental official course.

COMPULSIVE BEHAVIORS

My over the top inclinations began following the assault on our base

on June sixteenth. I was ill-equipped, out of uniform, and no rifle during a period of emergency. The evening of June seventeenth, I began spreading out my uniform with a specific goal in mind to get ready for the following assault. It was more than having my uniform close to my bed; it must be collapsed with a specific goal in mind and stacked in a specific request. My boots and glasses must be in a particular spot. Consistently, it's a good idea to have my uniform prepared in a battle climate; notwithstanding, that impulsive propensity proceeded subsequent to returning home. A long time after my organization, I actually return home from work and put my uniform on my washroom counter, all stacked and prepared, even on Friday evenings when I don't need to work during the weekend.

dditionally, my vehicle keys should be on the snare, my espresso is prepared to blend, and my lunch ready in the cooler. As a general rule, I am frequently excessively coordinated and controlled. I struggle when there are startling changes, as incapable to have lunch at 11 am, or I can't stop in my typical parking space. I say that I've my things prepared so I can unobtrusively leave the house, however I become upset assuming something is different.

To remunerate intellectually, I formed into a rendition of a moderate. I have under a case of individual things in my office and just a single conventional picture on my dividers. In accordance with my modesty, I don't have a divider with testaments and grants. My vehicle is for all intents and purposes void with the exception of the required things in the glove compartment and control center. I never have in excess of twelve messages in my inbox at work or my other email accounts. I have a couple of saved messages in consistent organizers and am just utilizing a minuscule level of my space assignment. It irritates me when things are forgotten about, or there is confusion, and I can't grasp how some collaborators have large number of messages in their inbox.

This moderate methodology has made me more productive. While turning into an official, my chiefs bored into our heads that it was smarter to be on schedule with 80% of the arrangement than being late with 100% of the arrangement on the grounds that no arrangement endures first contact. Armed force authority lectures that assuming you are ten minutes ahead of schedule, you are late. I have fostered a fixation on schedule. Our breeze up Howard Miller tolling divider clock that my significant other and I purchased on our first commemoration is a genuine fortune, and I find solace in hearing the rings like clockwork. Towards the finish of my sending, I changed from standard Casio type watches to Swiss watches with mechanical systems. Inside the initial two years, I overhauled my watches and got an incredible arrangement on an Omega Speedmaster Moon watch. This hand-wind watch is another fortune, and I wore this watch day by day for a really long time. After ten years, it was late for its

suggested support, so I changed to a pleasant Citizen watch with hands and nuclear time synchronization.

My time fixation isn't restricted to watches yet more in keeping a timetable. I put forth phenomenal attempts to ensure I am on schedule or right on time for everything. It is incredibly troublesome when a person or thing is late. It very well may be a straightforward thing as my girl's training, my better half getting back home after a gathering, preparing not beginning, or stand by in the specialist's office. At the point when individuals miss these time hacks, my pulse builds, my breaths become more limited, my chest fixes, and my brain begins hustling. I know there are intelligent explanations behind a large portion of these deferrals however have little command over the actual manifestations. My time fixation might be the reason I am getting a charge out of directing with my little girl's games since I can handle the clock.

PRESCRIPTIONS

My muscular specialist endorsed Tramadol for relief from discomfort for my proceeding with knee issues. He informed me that it was non-habit-forming and more grounded than Tylenol yet was not viewed as an opiate. I began the medicine by a couple of dosages daily, and I observed that the aggravation in my knee decreased. Following half a month on the medicine, I additionally observed that I partook in the somewhat high inclination, and it appeared to elevate my readiness and made me more engaged. I utilized this drug for quite a long time before my medical procedure and afterward again in the wake of minimizing from an OPIOID remedy. I expected to accept Tramadol as needed, up to a specific sum. I didn't take the medicine past the predetermined sum, and it immediately transformed into the daily practice to awaken, take a portion, on the other hand, the early in the day, after lunch and evening. Assuming I had a portion in the evening, I would experience difficulty getting to sleep.

I had persistent knee torment and extra medical procedures, so the Tramadol was not difficult to get. Nonetheless, at a certain point, my knee medical procedure recuperation didn't require additional prescriptions, so I halted. The withdrawal indications immediately began, and I had fretful a sleeping disorder for no less than three evenings. Fretfulness constrained me to rest in the extra room in the storm cellar so I would not keep my better half conscious, and afterward I was getting increasingly drained. By the fourth evening, I in the long run nodded off. Prior to another medical procedure, my muscular specialist again recommended Tramadol. I had the remedy filled and utilized it yet, however intentionally, I realized I ought not be on it that long as I had withdrawal indications already. This emphasis was a lot more limited, however I actually went through two evenings of withdrawal when I stopped.

I can envision how effectively it very well might be to mishandle lawful and illicit medications. I utilized Tramadol more than on a case by case basis, however I would not depict it as maltreatment as I utilized it inside as far as possible, and I acquired it legitimately from my muscular specialist. Inevitably of taking the medicine, I don't have the foggiest idea how viable it was for my knee torment, yet I exploited the slight high inclination. Concerning OPIOID solutions, I had just utilized the underlying portion and normally quit utilizing them before the primary remedy ran out. Narcotics had a higher inclination than Tramadol, yet they have caused sickness and clogging. Furthermore, I was unable to drive while taking OPIOIDs, and I was consistently anxious to have the option to drive again.

ALCOHOL

Alcohol is predominant inside our nearby society. Wisconsin is home to Miller Brewing Company, the Major League ball club is named "Brewers," and closely following with whelps and lager is standard before a Green Bay Packer football match-up or Milwaukee Brewers ball game. Wisconsin's punishment for a first-time frame driving while inebriated infringement is a misdeed while it is a crime in numerous different states. Experiencing childhood in my teen years, my folks provided me with a few beverages. I had a grasshopper at Christmas or a drink of blackberry cognac while deer hunting, yet I never went to parties or different spots with brew or alcohol.

One of the perspectives that I like with regards to Marquette University for school was that my support took me to the neighborhood VFW for pitchers of lager on my direction. My high level ordnance preparing in Fort Sill, I devoured a considerable amount of liquor at the clubs promptly off the post on our spend ends of the week. First year zeroed in on local gatherings on the ends of the week. One weekend, my support bought a jug of vodka and squeezed orange for two or three my companions and me. I don't recollect that evening by any means. I was oblivious and had no reaction to the security official's smelling salts when I returned to the residences, so I was moved by rescue vehicle to the nearby crisis office. I had the option to calm down enough with intravenous liquids, however that evening was not my best second and was exorbitant as I took care of the multitude of bills out of pocket.

My liquor utilize changed throughout the long term and a long time, alongside the sort of drink. Prior to arrangement, I for the most part burned-through lager, and after sending, I devoured red wine in view of the cell reinforcements and cholesterol benefits. Following a couple of years, I went to white wine since red wine would stain my teeth. I infrequently had hard alcohol in the house, and it was normally too much

work to blend a mixed drink, so I devoured it straight in more modest sums. I would commonly think about my utilization at the social level, yet it was quite often at home. I have not partaken in the bar scene since school, and I generally make a point about holding off on burning-through until I am agreed to the evening to try not to drive under the influence.

didn't think it was misuse since I didn't have headaches, and I didn't devour during the day or while at work. There have been periods when my utilization changed somewhat higher. Ordinarily, this would happen in the event that I was not locked in later in the evening, and it was a simple break to pump the brakes to me. I needn't bother with liquor, and there is no specific justification for why I have any. Maybe there is a little truth to the joke of fluid treatment, as that is my most probable explanation. Drinking is certifiably not a suggested method for dealing with stress as there are numerous hindering impacts. I was not careful on certain events and entered the inebriation stages. I was self centered and not contemplating my better half, little girl, and Molly.

EDICAL

I utilized a portion of my ailments as a support. I would purposely plan medical procedures to stay away from end of the week preparing or actual wellness tests. I additionally exploited the permitted debilitated leave for recuperation. I accomplished some work after the primary medical procedure or two and afterward went to marathon watching TV programs and deferred reacting to messages. In the spring of 2011, I encountered knee enlarging and extraordinary agony during my first outside run. Subsequent to checking on my MRI results, my PCP said I expected to alter my exercises to stretch my knee's life span because of my ligament harm. The Army gave me a long-lasting profile that limited me from running for the actual wellness test. The failure to run was a huge antagonistic change, as running has turned into my thing. I had lost my passionate reset, and I was a walker. A planned over two mile speed walk is approved rather than the two-mile run for those on profile. I had a proceeding with series of clinical issues throughout the long term that have brought about constraints. My knee caused agony and worry for a really long time, and I had eight tasks. My contrary foot has had a few issues and three medical procedures. With proceeded with torment, I can't genuinely run, I can't stoop on my right knee, nor would i be able to twist my knee enough to squat.

I lost one of my good ways of dealing with stress and had an increment in dissatisfaction with my proceeded with knee torment, and my actual availability and clinical issues added to discouragement sentiments. It regularly annoys me that I

can't get things done, and I need to be specific on what I can do, in any event, choosing if I would have the option to stroll around the state carnival for a couple of hours. I comprehend the tactical's prerequisite to have prepared and accessible powers. I support the perspective of isolating non-accessible staff. The military ought not keep work force who can't fill the fundamental roles. Assuming I had these equivalent ailments a couple of years prior, I would have likely been dependent upon clinical division. Be that as it may, the nearer you complete the full twenty years of dynamic assistance for retirement, the more you need to endure the aggravation and issues. I felt exceptionally exacting during this timeframe.

My clinical limits contrarily affected my cardiovascular exercises and gradually expanded my weight. The Army weight control program utilizes a screening interaction and muscle versus fat estimations to guarantee consistence. The screening system applies a singular's stature and weight against a sex and age graph to decide whether the individual requires a muscle versus fat estimation. In straightforward terms, in case the weight record is past the fitting age and sex, then, at that point, extra taping measures and recipes are utilized to decide a more explicit muscle versus fat estimation. For the principal half of my tactical profession, I would have the option to get on the scale in full uniform and still be well beneath the screening weight. Since my running limitation, and at last, my trekking limitation, my weight draws much nearer to the screening weight. I'm glad that I never surpassed the screening loads. I need to stay aware of the food sources I burn-through, however I do appreciate pizza and candy.

COMMUNICATION

Communication is a three-way road with basic paths of talking, tuning in, and grasping. I do well with tuning in and seeing, however I constantly battle with talking. Powerful correspondence can be a decent way of dealing with stress assuming each of the three paths are the correct way. In any case, correspondence is an all inclusive region that the vast majority can improve. During each assessment of my tactical activities, correspondence is consistently a region that surfaces for requiring improvement. Regularly, the right messages don't arrive at the planned party. I've considered issues with interchanges to be a kid by playing the phone game.

My greatest obstacle is the momentary seen judgment and aversion of discussion. As per human satisfying, I am worried about the possibility that that whoever I am talking with won't concur with my remarks, so I forgo speaking

out. I can work on my interchanges with almost everybody. I would not impart anything about my awful accidents to my significant other prior to composing First to Fire; along these lines, she didn't have the foggiest idea what, regardless, I encountered. I can unquestionably further develop correspondences with my administrator and associates, relatives, neighbors, and other school guardians. Someone can't help you assuming you don't express what's up. Someone can't uphold you in case you don't tell them happening.

HOBBIES

During both treatment medicines, my advisor prescribed going to a side interest. Enjoying a side interest that you appreciate will be a colossal positive method for dealing with stress. There are many side interests accessible to browse, and many individuals partake in their leisure activities and invest a lot of energy and cash on their side interests. A leisure activity can turn into a terrible way of dealing with stress contingent upon the choice of the side interest. For instance, assuming somebody has a fishing propensity, yet the person just goes fishing with a twelve-pack, that probably won't be a suitable hobby.

My difficulty is that I don't enjoy a leisure activity of interest. One of the side interests that I thought would be fun is gaming on the PlayStation. I tracked down a Playstation available to be purchased on Craigslist for under $100, and it accompanied a few invigorating games. Toward the start of my arrangement, one more US consultant got me snared on playing Call of Duty, a first-individual warfighting game-based fight in the European performance center of World War II. This Playstation accompanied a few forms of Call of Duty alongside a couple of other first-individual shooting match-ups. My significant other needed me to play these computer games when my girl was nowhere to be found, so my playing time was restricted. At the point when I played the games, I felt like I was getting upset from the subjects from the situations. I quit gaming, and my Playstation wound up sitting in our amusement community for a really long time. A large number of the games on Playstation, including warfighting or donning games, consume most of the day to load and play an emphasis or level. My family never observed interest in playing the sporting events on the Playstation. I observed the basic games on my iPad give an incredible mental interruption, immediately start and stop, and have no expanded uneasiness levels.

At the point when I was growing up, I had a radio-controlled vehicle that I delighted in, and I had an exorbitant interest in radio controlled toys. In the course of the most recent couple of years, I purchased a novice model of a helicopter and a plane, wanting to foster abilities to join a neighborhood radio-controlled plane club. Radio-controlled toys were an extremely fleeting and costly side interest. In the wake of expenditure more than $100 for the fledgling models, I had two or three endeavors at flight and smashed too often to the place of annihilation. I additionally understood that this was not the best side interest choice since it required a lot arranging and practice. The climate conditions must be practically great, the batteries completely energized, and I really wanted the accessible time. After this coordination and arranging, I would have the option to fly for under ten minutes before I smashed. I was self-trained and didn't have a companion or tutor to show me the nuts and bolts, and I believed that I would have the option to do rolls and circles like a semi-professional.

Many of the things that I appreciate don't fall into commonplace side interest classes. I appreciate home preparing our family suppers, trimming the grass, and chipping away at projects around the house. I partake in my little girl's games practices and games and going for Molly for a stroll. Most days, I appreciate driving my vehicle and the drive to work. I appreciate composing and composing on the PC. Innovation propels permitted me to compose or mess around on my iPad in the wake of driving my girl to her training, a mix of a few things I enjoy.

AND THE UGLY STIGMA

"PTSI isn't the individual declining to relinquish the past, yet the past declining to relinquish the individual." – Unknown

Stigma surrounds the invisible injury aspects of PTSI. It is easy to have compassion for a soldier with a missing arm coming home from deployment, but there are no obvious visible signs for a soldier with PTSI returning from arrangement. Not exclusively is PTSI undetectable, however it will likewise differ significantly starting with one individual then onto the next. Individual triggers and remembering the occasion might be unique, responses and evasions might be changed, and treatment might be unique. The overall impression of a veteran with PTSD is that of a male that is logical mishandling liquor and drugs and most likely has murderous or self-destructive inclinations. A Google® picture look for "veteran PTSD" will result in various photographs of white guys in an Army uniform looking discouraged by twisting around with their hands on their heads.

There is even an animation picture in the outcomes that portrays a devoted regular citizen expressing, "Incredible to have you home, Bro! Also NOT a scratch on you… " remaining close to a male in uniform with "PTSD" for his name tape and a ticking explosive for his head. Current media rushes to recognize earlier military assistance for mass shooting suspects, which may subliminally interface PTSD with these superfluous and terrible events.

he shortened form of PTSD is normal yet explained as posttraumatic stress issue have extra undertones. The American Psychiatric Association formalized the term posttraumatic stress problem in 1980 as an emotional wellness condition. The customs permitted analyze, research, treatment, protection, and handicap benefits. Notwithstanding, the problem angles suggest previous conditions, though injury includes harm at a certain

point. It is trying to remember somebody with PTSI as the individual doesn't have noticeable signs, similar to an arm sling or a wheelchair. Others are bound to assist somebody with noticeable indications of a physical issue. At the point when I was recuperating from my knee medical procedure, others asked what occurred and offered assistance by opening entryways and conveying things. My bosses gave incredible mercy permitting improvement leave and downtime for follow up arrangements. My interior convictions that in the event that I express anything about PTSI that it would require support, and nobody would get what I have experienced in light of the fact that they were not there. Looking for treatment for a physical issue that happened is more normal than looking for treatment for an issue that might be seen as a weakness.

Typical wounds are perceived and respected in everyday society and inside the military. Frequently, I will see an image of an assistance part with consume wounds or removal and a remark about sharing and preferring the photograph to foster help and mindfulness. For military staff, the Purple Heart is the most seasoned military honor. It is entitled for those injured or killed in any activity against a foe of the United States or because of a demonstration of any such adversary or contradicting military. Regardless of previous President Bush's comments and endeavors to eliminate the shame, the models state unequivocally that posttraumatic stress issue doesn't fit the bill for a Purple Heart. I'm personally acquainted with people with expanded honors, including the Purple Heart, and others that never gotten the suitable honors. Shockingly, a few people go past extraordinary lengths to make themselves search useful for individual gain.

There are a lot of legitimate instances of PTSI, and tragically, there are individuals who exploit the circumstance. Military incapacity installments are charge absolved and are reliant upon the level of handicap appraisals, and PTSI can have a huge rating. Since PTSI is an undetectable physical issue, it very well might be enticing for certain people to swindle. Notwithstanding, the Department of Veterans Affairs doesn't give inability remuneration dependent on the actual analysis, yet on the seriousness of the indications on every day social and work life. The Department of Veterans Affairs perceives PTSI for a help associated handicap however puts the weight on the veteran to finish structures and extra reports for approval. Remuneration for posttraumatic stress is gathered with other emotional wellness conditions, like schizophrenia, uneasiness, discouragement, and bipolar issues. The gathering of mental issues has a full scope of handicap appraisals, while numerous other ailments have restrictions. A 0% rating

would be suitable for a determination, and the manifestations don't meddle with word related and social capacities. In examination, 100% would be reasonable for all out word related and social hindrance with terribly improper conduct and confusion to put and time.

Realizing that something wasn't right and that I was impacted by PTSI was a lethargic interaction. It was for a considerable length of time and required numerous months to sort out what was off-base. Besides, when I understood that something was wrong, I believed I expected to conceal it so nobody could discover. I was humiliated that I struggled managing a few occasions from my arrangement years prior. Not exclusively was it from quite a while in the past, no one knew what I went through or experienced. My organization was one of a kind, and no one had similar encounters, and I sent without the standard unit support. The recognizable picture of a veteran with PTSI is savagery, outrage, fury, and irritable. I'm the direct inverse. I can't recollect the last time I shouted out of resentment at anybody. I have not hit or harmed anybody, and I have not tossed an espresso cup across the kitchen. I had been enraged or disappointed, yet I suppressed the sentiments. Upon conflict, I escape or submit, which are probable not the best responses.

I was reluctant to tell anyone that I was going to treatment and getting treatment. In the first place, there was a shallow degree of trust with anybody at work. I sought places of expanded liabilities and advancement openings and was anxious about the possibility that that I would be considered to be more vulnerable and not intellectually extreme. I planned treatment arrangements in the early evening, so I would just need to go home somewhat early and still return home near my standard time. During my recuperation time from knee and foot activities, I had treatment, so I could say I was going to treatment with the feeling that it was exercise based recuperation. I caught a few discussions concerning how a few troopers blamed PTSI and some other unfriendly discernments, so I was exceptionally wary so no one would know about my issues.

ore than saw as a shortcoming, PTSI can make vulnerability about proceeded with military assistance. As a tactical assistance part, I have an obligation to remain medicinally prepared and accessible. Assuming I am harmed, I should illuminate the military and look for treatment to improve. Assuming that a physical issue happens, you need to recuperate adequately to be prepared and accessible once more; nonetheless, in case the injury is sufficiently serious or can't completely recuperate, the assistance part will go through a clinical board process and perhaps medicinally isolated. Since a genuine finding of PTSI needs somewhere around a month with

manifestations, realizing that side effects fluctuate in seriousness and practicality, and there is no closure state, it makes illuminating the military undeniably challenging, particularly assuming it might bring about partition. The conceivable clinical detachment persuades you to attempt to adapt all alone. There are added difficulties to the extensive medical care is I had military clinical records and private clinical records, and the two arrangements of documents don't combine. Separate record-keeping might bring about duplication or an absence of coordination. In a functioning military status, the military gave my medical services. Since I was outside of the space of a tactical medical clinic, I had the option to utilize neighborhood network specialists. The military paid the neighborhood specialists. All things considered, the wellbeing records stayed with the neighborhood specialist, and I would need to give set up approval to impart portions of these accounts to the military. Armed force guidelines require the assistance individuals to uncover wounds and ailments to their unit as it might influence status. This necessity is generally simplefor a compound fracturedleg; however, this is much more muddled with revealing PTSI. The impacted individual will initially need to comprehend that they have PTSI. It took me a while to converse with somebody about my manifestations, which was a very long time after my organization. An individual should have indications for somewhere around a month prior to a specialist can make a finding, and the seriousness and kind of manifestations will differ. There is no limit for announcing, so an assistance part might have the attentiveness to report when they understand they are impacted with manifestations, upon conclusion, during treatment, utilizing prescriptions, or other methods for dealing with stress. It is for the most part testing to concede issues; in this way, there is a higher probability to postpone reporting.

needed to keep away from the appearance that I was getting on board with that temporary fad and attempting to exploit the framework. It required very nearly nine years to begin understanding the impacts of PTSI and choosing to converse with somebody about this issue. I began understanding the effects in 2015 preceding I had musings of leaving the tactical help. In 2015, I had around 15 years of dynamic assistance and would require no less than five additional to fit the bill for retirement. The evasion of the fad was a part of not discussing the negative parts of my organization. Toward the start of 2018, I was reluctant to start pharmacology treatment since it might bring up issues of accessibility to convey. My tactical health care coverage kept up with my remedy records, yet never hailed me in a framework for emotional wellness concerns. In 2018, I went through a trooper preparation cycle and clinical screening to guarantee accessibility. Sertraline was on my rundown of current meds, so I had an extra stop with the military social wellbeing trained professionals. His anxiety was making sure

that the treatment was what I thought I needed.

During my treatment meetings, I reclassified my meaning of administration. Regularly in the military, there are assumptions, and we put out up those objectives dependent on those assumptions. An assumption is that I am an Army official, so I ought to endeavor to be an administrator of an organization and a brigade. Particularly being in a functioning status, there should be an issue assuming I am not an administrator. Envision Lieutenant Colonel Hal Moore from We Were Soldiers as the unwritten assumption for an authority. I pondered my activities during a portion of my unpleasant occasions, and I didn't make the authority like moves. During the side of the road bomb assault, I remained in the firearm truck and watched, and during the assault on the Afghan Police station, I was the senior official, and everything I did was drive the weapon truck. I set the bar high for anticipated norms, and I didn't meet these objectives, and I beat myself okay with missing the mark. Maybe the military isn't the best profession decision now in my life, and that is OK since I actually am a decent pioneer by setting the model and persuading individuals towards a typical goal.

I didn't plan to begin composing a book when I composed First to Fire. My advisor urged me to expound on my horrible mishaps during PTSI directing. From the beginning, it was a couple of conventional, short sentences with several trendy expression feelings. As directing advanced, I was urged to compose more subtleties, which brought about several brief tales about my two horrible mishaps. As I was composing, I thought that it is more straightforward to open up and be straightforward. Composing additionally gave the chance to share my story. I have not imparted my story to anybody, including my significant other and little girl. I wanted to catch my notes and pictures to have my girl have a superior comprehension of what I went through.

While composing has been restorative, it has likewise made a few tensions. To keep on advancing through treatment and increment my confidence, I realized I needed to deliver my story public. I dealt with the arrangement that my story is accessible to anybody, causing you to feel uncovered and living in an air pocket. More tensions emerged soon after distribution. I utilized online media to report my arrangement story on Amazon®. I got a request from our public issues office showing they needed to distribute an article about me and my composition. They gave a poll that contained straightforward inquiries: what's going on with the book and why I composed it. I was straightforward in my replies, and I had demonstrated that composing had begun through PTSI guiding with consolation from my therapist.

My significant other gave me a mindful warning to ensure I knew what I was getting into when I delivered my book. She was worried that I had just barely imparted my story to her as she read the drafts, and presently I was distributing so that anybody might see. Anybody would have the option to peruse my accounts, and individuals should converse with me about them. With the public issues news discharge, it referenced that I began composing my book on account of the consolation of my specialist to expound on my horrendous accidents. Nearby media (The Oconomowoc Enterprise paper, The Waukesha Freeman paper, WSAU Wausau radio broadcast, and TMJ4 Milwaukee TV slot) centered their tale regarding how composing helped for PTSI. With assent, TMJ4 composed a meeting with my advisor to give an expert assessment on how composing benefited me.

t was trying to acknowledge that I had PTSI however was significantly more testing to openly recognize that I had PTSI, particularly for certain loved ones. I feared what others would consider me or how others would treat me. I had bipolar sentiments after delivering my story. Some portion of me was eager to advance my book as it was a huge accomplishment, and I was restless to share my story since I realized it was not the same as the vast majority of individuals that I knew, and nobody knew my entire story. I had expected to a greater degree a reaction. The input I got was, "I perused your book, and it was great." I based my response to a ridiculous assumption that individuals will drop what they are doing to peruse my story.

The media requests zeroed in on the PTSI parts of my story; nonetheless, no one has posed inquiries about my arrangement nor the PTSI issues. I either composed the ideal book with no follow-on conversation or questions, or individuals are reluctant to converse with me about it. I think individuals are terrified to discuss it. Since the time I came out with the PTSI mark as beginning to compose my book, no one has inquired as to whether I was doing approve or said anything regarding it. PTSI isn't infectious and noticeable as a pink eye. I don't want an inside and out philosophical conversation, yet some close to home registration would be appreciated.

The "deal with it" disposition that some have towards those with PTSI impacts the shame. For instance, after a prospective employee meeting, I was educated that I was not sure, and I absolutely should have been more ready. PTSI isn't a condition that one can "deal with it." I was prepared for that meeting yet had zero command over my limited focus, expanded pulse, and other nervousness side effects. Concerning shame, this is incomprehensible from which an individual can't escape due to various guidelines or restrictions. PTSI is an

undetectable injury, so a questioner may not see any signs, and it would be abnormal to go into a meeting and report that you have PTSI. There would almost certainly be a two-section reaction – first, in case one can't deal with a basic gathering, how might he/she handle this work, and second – assuming there is a repudiating of PTSI toward the start of the meeting, does he/she fulfill the clinical maintenance guidelines? In regular citizen business circumstances, the American Disabilities Act might give some insurance, however having a physical issue in the military has the chance of separation.

There is a discernment that in case I were more occupied and more connected with, I would not choose not to move on. In the course of recent years, I had additional time to burn and could perhaps be more occupied. I would sit in the grandstands without help from anyone else at swim practice for 90 minutes as it was not reasonable to be driving this way and that. In any case, since I would be more occupied would not imply that undesirable musings would stop. The undesirable considerations would come at practically any season of day and not just when I was bored.

I feel awkward when outsiders approach me to say thanks to me for my administration. I go to work and back home again in my uniform, and I make not many stops, generally just for gas. Either in the lift at the specialist's center or the service station, a more bizarre will move toward me and say thanks to me for my administration. I know it's benevolent; nonetheless, it seems like bogus satisfaction. It appears to be unconventional that a more abnormal says thanks to me for going about my business, and they have no clue about what I do for sure I have done. The common, "Thank you for your administration," remarks are cover proclamations simply because I am wearing my work outfit. You don't see outsiders going to a technician in face cloths at the supermarket coming back from work and saying thanks to them for their service.

MORAL INJURIES

"Moral Injury is separated from PTSI in that it straightforwardly identifies with culpability and disgrace veterans experience because of submitting activities that conflict with their ethical codes." – Chuck Norris

There is a difference between moral injury and PTSI, although they are similar. The Department of Veterans Affairs defines PTSI as a "mental disorder that requires a medical diagnosis" and moral injury as a "dimensional issue." An ethical physical issue is the point at which it has abused an inner voice profound conviction. The idea of moral injury can be followed back to Cain and Abel in Genesis, Chapter 4. After Cain kills Abel, God marks Cain so others won't kill him. At the point when an ethical physical issue happens when killing is essential or difficult to stay away from, an individual is always showed signs of change, everlastingly set apart by their activities. Moral injury isn't as of now a perceived clinical injury, yet it can impact an individual's conduct. Moral injury might exist together with PTSI however requires separate distinguishing proof and treatment. PTSI can truly and mentally influence an individual, while an ethical physical issue is a contention between a solid, individual conviction against an action.

Just as PTSI has various levels of seriousness, and the side effects can change, moral injury is variable. I was an immediate observer to some problematic moral exercises on organization. I didn't effectively partake in these problematic moral exercises, yet I never really prevented them from occurring. For instance, when we went on watches, the neighborhood Afghan children were not generally eager to see us. Regularly, more youthful young men would toss golf ball-sized rocks at the heavy armament specialist on top of the vehicle. The young men tossed stones at the heavy armament specialist in hostility and acted like a potential physical issue, and terminating the automatic rifle in counter would not be suitable. There was a need to react to show that the children should quit tossing the stones; any other way, they would continue to toss. In this way, the heavy weapons specialist ordinarily had a little modest bunch of grape-sized rocks to toss stones back at the young men. I didn't toss rocks, yet I had a stone heap in the turret while I was a heavy weapons specialist. This reaction was viewed as proper by the heavy armament specialists and nearby US counsels, yet the standing principles of commitment didn't support this activity, nor was it legitimately responsible.

Wild canines introduced an issue around the neighborhoods they were horrible and conveyed various sicknesses. To lessen the issue, a little gathering of US guides would lure the wild canines quickly outside of the fence. The little gathering utilized their guns and rifles and fired the wild canines. This interaction transformed into a rivalry, and it appeared to be a game. I didn't go with the gathering to take shots at the wild canines, however I said nothing regarding it. In both of these exercises, it was a way to the outcome, yet all at once possible not moral or legitimate. Notwithstanding, the young men tossing rocks and wild canines introduced a risk, yet I didn't have a superior solution.

While not selective, most upright wounds include demise or injury. I had a discussion with an Army Chaplain in regards to the effect of moral injury among Soldiers. The Chaplain depicted a story where the help part was the heavy weapons specialist on a firearm truck going through a hazardous piece of an Iraq city. A kid stepped before his folks and lit a hand crafted bomb and began a tossing movement towards the weapon truck when the assistance part drew in the kid with the assault rifle. Not exclusively was the kid probably momentarily killed, yet the custom made bomb arrived on him. This assistance part's fundamental concern was assuming God planned to pardon him. The Chaplain further expressed that the Lord's instruction is "Thou will not kill," ought to be renamed into murder, and there is a distinction among killing and murder and the goals behind those activities. There is a critical contrast between an individual shooting somebody to take their vehicle as opposed to shooting somebody attempting to kill you or your kindred colleagues for assurance. While the subsequent demise of somebody is something very similar in these occasions, the inspiration and plan are opposites.

The most common type of moral injury is from battle and inclusion with death or killing. In any case, individuals can experience the ill effects of not making a move outside of battle. An individual might observer the prompt result of a serious auto crash. While genuinely ready to go back and forth back

to the scene and render help, they forge ahead their way some place and don't need the burden of making a difference. At that point, he/she might believe that others will pause and help, however they might see a news report later on with regards to how sad the mishap was, and wounded their inward heart since they realized they ought to have made a difference. Moral injury isn't restricted to those that pull the trigger. Authorities and activities work force who approve assaults, airstrikes or ordnance might confront moral wounds for the impacts of the inadvertent blow-back. A military pilot could have the right bomb and right area of the objective. In any case, the objective knowledge could be off-base, and the military pilot could experience the ill effects of moral injury from the passings from his/her bombs, despite the fact that he/she didn't do anything actually illegal.

a definitive motivation behind the military is to overcome the adversary to ensure the US. The demonstration of killing is innate inside the calling as long for what it's worth against the adversary while protecting oneself, their association, the guiltless individuals of the far off country, or individuals of the US. Demise from battle activities ought not bring about moral injury except if there are unexpected blunders. Inadvertent mistakes might be blow-back from bombs or somebody not revealing ill-advised cross examination strategies. There isn't a limit for the presence of moral injury as it is a dimensional problem.

I relate to two minor moral wounds from my sending. My first upright battle is the ordnance mission that I determined on October 22nd, 2006, which brought about ten setbacks. I discovered a little while later that this counter-fire mission brought about ten setbacks. As far as anyone knows, the assault helicopters radioed the fight harm appraisal to the tasks place subsequent to showing up back in the space when we quit terminating. As I determined the gunnery part of the mission, I played a huge part that brought about those losses. It is great to realize that I had the option to utilize my field cannons abilities in battle that had results. Amusingly, this gunnery mission was one of the features of my sending yet brought about a few setbacks. For this ordnance mission, our bases got approaching rocket flames, and we reacted by terminating gunnery back to the rocket dispatch site. We reacted with ordnance to stop the capability of their rockets from making losses of ourselves. The fight harm evaluation demonstrated ten losses. Ten people harmed or killed, and fundamentally impacted their families as they were children, spouses, and fathers.

illing and causing deliberate damage conflicts with Christian convictions. I feel defended in my activities and terminating gunnery in light of the approaching rockets.

Teamwork and actual distance decreased the effect of these setbacks. Many individuals are engaged with terminating exact mounted guns shoot. Spectators should have the option to distinguish the objective and make redresses. A few people need to get the objective data, process the information, and send the guidelines to the howitzer team. Howitzer teams ordinarily need something like six people to emplace the firearm, load the ammo and unequivocally point the cannon tube. One individual can't fire exact ordnance fires as it is a common obligation among a group of people, and every individual should be exact and proficient at their particular employment obligations. Dave Grossman portrays the mental effect of actual distance in his book On Killing: The Psychological Cost of Learning to Kill in War and Society (1995). The actual vicinity to killing is the fundamental variable for how effective the occasion will be for the individual. In case you can't see the killing (plane pilots, mounted guns, maritime rockets), there is less effect on an individual than a nearby, private execution (hand-to-hand, blade, gun). At the point when I determined the gunnery for this ordnance mission, I was in a shut room a couple of miles away, and I saw just guides and diagrams. I could undoubtedly hear and feel the howitzer terminating, however I was unable to hear the round impacts nor any destruction.

Another minor moral injury that I endured was during a brief firefight. One more US consultant and I went on an exceptionally perplexing night perception mission with various imprudences. Not long after 12 PM, on the fifth commemoration of the 9/11 assaults, our position lit getting little arms fire from AK-47s on our right side. I was a heavy weapons specialist on the truck, and the other US guide was the driver. I have nitty gritty notes on this mission up to the place of assault. There are two spots where I demonstrated that I discharged the assault rifle, yet there was no note on my every day schedule. The uncommon part is that I don't have a reasonable picture to me of my responses upon attack.

I had an adrenaline surge toward the beginning of the assault on the grounds that my memory skips around for some time. I don't absolutely know the foe area or the quantity of adversary staff. I realized that there were a couple of Afghan Soldiers on our right-hand side of our perception point who beginning going around and bringing fire back. I don't think I terminated at the foe since I didn't have the foggiest idea about their area. The Afghan Soldiers would have been before the foe, so I more likely than not discharged overhead for suppressive shoot, which is discharging our weapons in the adversary's overall course to have them quit shooting at us, making them look for cover. With the developing dissatisfaction that evening with the various imprudences and the unexpected adrenaline surge, I more likely than not happened limited focus as my

recollections upon assault beginning are in short spurts.

It is wistful realizing that I shot an automatic weapon in a firefight on the fifth commemoration of 9/11, yet it annoys me as I can't unmistakably recall the entire evening. I can't remember whether I inclined down to point with the sights or then again in the event that I pointed the automatic rifle the overall overhead way. Joined with the obscurity, foe discharging, and Afghan Soldiers shooting, I have no clue about where my shots went. There were no losses or wounds, so no one in the prompt area was shot. I couldn't say whether my slugs hit the close by mud-walled house, hit a sheep in a herd a pretty far, or affected honestly in the soil. My ethical battle is the questions; explicitly, I don't have the foggiest idea where the rounds impacted.

I learned of the big guns results a little while after the occasion dependent on noise data. As I found out with regards to the outcomes, I saw the report that demonstrated ten foe losses. In military phrasing, a setback can be a physical issue or a casualty. I couldn't say whether the setbacks in our cannons mission were harmed, killed, or a mix. I was not a subject of an examination in the two circumstances, so I can expect there were no accidental mistakes. In any case, I can't say the big guns adjusts or the shots were not blunder free. I left the gunnery base inside about fourteen days of the counter-shoot mission and lost situational attention to that space. It took over a month to discover that the mission had losses, and I never found a non military personnel setback objection. Cannons is a region weapon, implying that sway region is enormous, and each round affecting won't land in a similar spot. The point in this fire mission was the rocket's beginning area, and our big guns adjusts affected all around this particular point. Ten setbacks appear to be high as it doesn't take that many individuals to fire rockets. I would not know whether there were various rocket groups, assuming the adversary was preparing initiates, or then again in case a portion of the losses were close by civilians.

The honest inquiry that regular citizen people pose to a tactical veteran, "Did you kill anybody?" is upsetting for me to reply. While I didn't discharge my rifle and fire somebody, I added to the mounted guns mission with ten setbacks. I didn't observer passing, however I helped cause it. It is a peculiar feeling of achievement yet not something to brag about, particularly since I don't have a clue about the particular setback status. I need to say that I helped the tactical mission by lessening the foe. While actually, I added to ten setbacks, I have passionate faltering recognizing the facts.

The manifestations or delayed consequences of moral injury are regularly disgracing, guilt,

and outrage. Be that as it may, as PTSI, moral injury and its manifestations are extremely individualistic. There is an absence of examination on moral injury, particularly the treatment of the ethical injury. The Department of Veteran Affairs is trying an intercession called Impact of Killing in War, which can be finished in six meetings. It is an altered intellectual treatment that spotlights on training, ID of intellectual attributions, self-absolution, and setting things right. Since moral injury is soul and religious, pastors, and the strict local area can give the most advantageous treatments.

CHARLIE MIKE

"Today was great. Today was enjoyable. Tomorrow is another." –

Dr. Seuss

Charlie Mike is military vernacular for continue mission, with the military phonetic alphabet letters for C and M, which is often the abbreviation for continue mission. Living with and managing PTSI is a Charlie Mike. I accomplished and took in an enormous sum in my 27 years of military assistance. Notwithstanding my extremely interesting organization experience, I formed and improved myself into an empathetic individual. The Army ingrained and built up numerous extraordinary morals and qualities, similar to honesty, regard, obligation, and honor. The Army Ethics diagrams my convictions on how I served and why I served. I served for the love of the nation and to safeguard the American public and qualities. I presented with character, successfully and effectively. The Lord's charges are settled with my solid uprightness to treat individuals decently and make the right decision and legal.

he military gave freedoms to accomplish my Masters of Business Management degree and my Professional Human Resource accreditation for proficient qualifications. Finishing various military schools all through my vocation showed me elusive subjects, similar to mission achievement, cooperation, research, and strategic and innovative information in endless regions. I learned authority characteristics in getting sorted out collaborations towards a shared objective. I figured out how to persuade, assess, and commit the proper assets. The military gave me freedoms to see regions of the planet, from the Far East to the Mid-East and Europe. I had freedoms to see many pieces of our extraordinary Nation, from the Pacific Northwest to the Nation's capital. I acquired viewpoint on the world, public, state, and local

legislatures and techniques. My variety expanded, and my social mindfulness developed. The Army weight control program and actual wellness prerequisites assisted me with keeping a sound way of life. I got quality medical care when I caused injury or sickness, and the military gave quality medical services to my family.

o one will have the chances or encounters that the military gave me in the course of the last 25 years. Who else can say that they have been in a passage under the Korean Demilitarized Zone, partaken in a Dunkel Weiss in a lager garden in Germany, discharged howitzer guns, fired rockets, drove huge trucks and followed vehicles, shot weapons in battle, or had chai tea with an Afghan senior? All through my tactical profession, I had nice remuneration, benefits, medical care, and employer stability. I'm appreciative that I had my sending encounters and surprisingly more thankful to have endure them. In basically every cycle model, the last advance is assessing. For any improvement, it is basic to have a legitimate assessment to figure out what works and what doesn't. Going through my battle encounters and going through treatment, I have a sensible assessment of me. I found out with regards to myself and PTSI, what it has meant for me, and what works for myself and what doesn't. Posttraumatic stress is a physical issue and should be considered to be a physical issue rather than an issue. This view will keep on breaking the disgrace, and perhaps others languishing will be more open over help.

The Department of Veterans Affairs clinical offices give general medical care, and they have therapy programs for mental and medical problems, including PTSI. The Department of Veterans Affairs clinical focuses are standard emergency clinics that give clinical treatment to veterans. There are explicit models to be qualified for the Department of Veterans Affairs clinical focus administrations. It by and large requires an assistance associated injury or inability; subsequently, PTSI would require documentation, and the veteran enlisted. In case a tactical assistance individual served in a disaster area, they could get rearrangement directing from the Department of Veterans Affairs Vet Centers. Vet Centers are local area based advising focuses that give a wide scope of social and mental administrations, including proficient correction guiding to Veterans and families. Clinical specialists might have the option to give treatment or references, and non military personnel authorized advisors with PTSI preparing can give guiding treatment.

Understanding and looking for help are the initial phases in the treatment of PTSI. Have the individual mental fortitude to request help on the off chance that you want it. The

Department of Veterans Affairs and the tactical administrations are broadening assets and projects, however the most significant agreement is close to home. Consistently, I got a self destruction anticipation instructions to get familiar with a portion of the signs and assets for help. I discovered that the self destruction rate among veterans is 22%, and I was aware of several generic casualties. During a new self destruction instructions, the primary half was the common PowerPoint slides. Then, at that point, an all around regarded, extremely senior pioneer stood up and recounted their story and how they were promptly after an endeavor. The companion interceded, and the mate took the senior chief to the crisis office for help. I knew this senior chief and their companion for quite some time, and I was stunned to hear their story.

After numerous months, I get what works best to deal with my indications and realize that it is a mix of a few reasonable instruments. I realize that I want to keep on zeroing in on the fitting devices, and these may require minor changes now and again. A portion of the deficient systems, like remedies and liquor, are more straightforward to change and stay away from, and a few, like withdrawal and over the top propensities, will require nonstop endeavors of progress. I understand that I was inside changed everlastingly, medicines will improve dealing with the manifestations, and I may never be completely healed.

Maintain perspective.

"Don't pass judgment on individuals. You don't have the foggiest idea what sort of fight they are fighting."

"One man's junk is another man's fortune."

"Don't yuck others' yums."

There are numerous truisms and citations to advise us that individuals have alternate points of view. There is an animation that portrays an individual on the left noticing a sideways "6" and an individual on the right that is contending that it is a "9." Both people are right as it is reliant upon their viewpoint. Others can assist those with PTSI by consolation and uphold and can dive deeper into this injury to assist with breaking the disgrace. There are monstrous missions, associations, and organizations carrying more attention to finding support. PTSI is an exceptionally individualistic physical issue, and backing might arrive in an assortment of structures. The most effective help can be studying PTSI and what it means for individuals. Open correspondence is fundamental. Tuning in, comprehension, and backing will go far.

www.ingramcontent.com/pod-product-compliance
Lightning Source LLC
LaVergne TN
LVHW041058150826
845673LV00007B/1827

* 9 7 9 8 7 7 9 7 2 2 3 1 5 *